Fundamentals of Neurophysiology

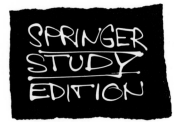

Fundamentals of
Neurophysiology

edited by

ROBERT F. SCHMIDT

with contributions by

JOSEF DUDEL

WILFRID JÄNIG

ROBERT F. SCHMIDT

MANFRED ZIMMERMANN

translated by Derek Jordan and Inge Jordan

 SPRINGER-VERLAG

New York   Heidelberg   Berlin   1975

Robert F. Schmidt
Physiologisches Institut der Universität Kiel
2300 Kiel
Olshausenstrasse 40/60
West Germany

Josef Dudel
Physiologisches Institut der Technischen
Universität München
8000 München 80
Ismaningerstrasse 19
West Germany

Wilfrid Jänig
Physiologisches Institut der Universität Kiel
2300 Kiel
Olshausenstrasse 40/60
West Germany

Manfred Zimmermann
II. Physiologisches Institut der Universität Heidelberg
6900 Heidelberg
Im Neuenheimer Feld 326
West Germany

Library of Congress Cataloging in Publication Data

Schmidt, Robert F.
    Fundamentals of neurophysiology.

    Translation of Grundriss der Neurophysiologie, 3rd edition
    Bibliography: p.
    1.Neurophysiology. I.Title.
    [DNLM: 1.Neurophyiology. WL102 G889]
    QP361.S3213   612'.8   74-18500

ISBN 0–387–06871–6 Springer-Verlag New York Heidelberg Berlin
ISBN 3–540–06871–6 Springer-Verlag Berlin Heidelberg New York

PREFACE

The English edition of this book has been prepared from the third German edition published in December 1974. The first two German editions, published in 1971 and 1972, respectively, were very well received in Germany. We hope that this English version will enjoy a similar popularity by students wishing to understand the essential concepts relevant to the fascinating field of neurophysiology.

The evolution of this book has been unique. The first edition was based on a series of lectures presented for many years to first-year physiology students at the Universities of Heidelberg and Mannheim. These lectures were converted into a series of 38 programmed texts, and after extensive testing, published as a programmed textbook of neurophysiology (Neurophysiologie programmiert, Springer-Verlag Heidelberg, 1971). Thereafter the present text was written and thoroughly brought up to date. Throughout this period all of the authors were members of the Department of Physiology in Heidelberg allowing for maximum cooperation at all stages of this endeavor.

With regard to the English edition, I wish to express my appreciation to Mr. Derek Jordan and Mrs. Inge Jordan for translating this book, and to my colleagues Dr. Mark Rowe and Dr. Dean O. Smith for their valuable comments and suggestions on the English manuscript. I express my grateful thanks to the publishers, both in Heidelberg and New York, for their unfailing courtesy and for their extraordinary efficiency.

Kiel, Germany, 1975   ROBERT F. SCHMIDT

v

CONTENTS

Fundamentals of Neurophysiology

1

THE STRUCTURE OF
THE NERVOUS SYSTEM

1.1 The Nerve Cells

Neurons. The building blocks of the nervous system are the *nerve cells*, which are also called *ganglion cells* but usually referred to as *neurons*. It is estimated that the human brain possesses 25 billion cells. Like all animal cells, each neuron is bounded by a cell membrane that encloses the contents of the cell, that is, the cytoplasm (cell fluid) and the nucleus. The size and shape of these neurons fluctuate widely, but the structural plan is always the same (Fig. 1-1): a cell body, or *soma*, and the processes from this cell body, namely, an *axon* (neurite) and usually several *dendrites*. The neuron shown in diagrammatic form in Fig. 1-1 has one axon and four dendrites. The axon and the dendrites normally divide into a varying number of branches (collaterals) after emerging from the soma.

The classification of the neuronal processes into an axon and several dendrites is made on the basis of *function*: the axon links the nerve cell with other cells. The axons of other neurons terminate on the dendrites and also on the soma. In order to make sure that you know the three important terms—soma, axon, and dendrite—draw Fig. 1-2 on a sheet of paper and give the correct names of the various parts indicated by the letters *a* to *g*. The answers are given on page 277, where the key to all the exercises begins.

Figure 1-3 illustrates various types of neurons. Notice in particular the great variation in the dendritic formations. Some neurons, for

Note: In this chapter a brief anatomical-histological introduction to the structure of the nervous system is given. These introductory remarks are intended only for students who have no previous knowledge of neuroanatomy. Anyone possessing such knowledge should check it immediately by working through test questions Q 1.1 to 1.5 on page 5, Q 1.6 on page 7, Q 1.7 to 1.9 on page 10, and Q 1.10 to 1.14 on page 15; and then continue with Chapter 2.

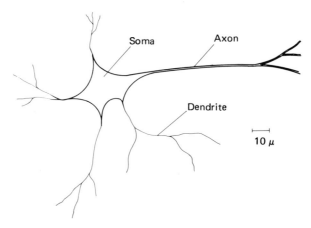

Fig. 1-1. Schematic diagram of a neuron showing the names of the various parts of the cell. The scale is intended to give an indication of the approximate dimensions.

example, neuron c, possess profusely branched dendrites, but in others, for example, neurons a and b, the ratio of soma surface to dendrite surface is somewhat more balanced. Finally, there are also neurons (d, e) that have no dendrites. The diameter of the neuronal cell bodies is in the order of magnitude of 5 to 100 μ (1 mm = 1,000 μ). The dendrites can be several hundred microns long.

As can be seen from the illustrations, one axon (synonyms: neurite, axon cylinder, axis cylinder) originates in each case from the soma of every neuron. This axon then usually splits up into branches called *collaterals*. The axons vary greatly in length. Often they are only a few microns long, but occasionally, for example, in the case of certain neurons in humans and other large mammals, they are much more than a meter long (for more details see Sec. 3 of this chapter).

Synapses. As already mentioned, the axon and all its collaterals join the nerve cell with other cells, which can be other nerve cells,

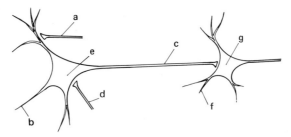

Fig. 1-2. Schematic diagram of two neurons. Give the names of the parts of the cells indicated by letters *a* to *g* (see text).

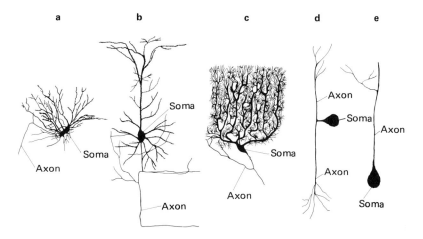

Fig. 1-3. Examples of the variety of shapes of neurons. See text for discussion. (After Ramon y Cajal.)

muscle cells, or glandular cells. The *junction of an axonal ending with other cells is called a synapse.* Figure 1-4 shows examples of neuronal junctions. If an axon or an axon collateral ends on the soma of another neuron, then we speak of an *axo-somatic synapse.* Correspondingly, a synapse between an axon and a dendrite is called an *axo-dendritic* synapse, and a synapse between two axons is called an *axo-axonic* synapse. If an axon ends on a skeletal muscle fiber, then this particular synapse is called a *neuromuscular end plate* (see Fig. 3-2). Synapses on muscle fibers of the intestines (smooth muscles) and on glandular cells have no special names.

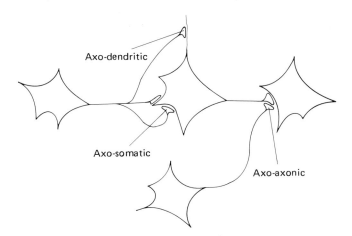

Fig. 1-4. Schematic diagram of synapses. See text for discussion.

Effectors. So far, we have learned that the nervous system is composed of individual cells called neurons. Most neurons are connected by synapses to other neurons to form neuronal circuits. However, the axons of a small number of neurons do not contact other neurons but, instead, connect with muscle cells or glandular cells. The striated skeletal muscles, the smooth muscles of the intestines, and the glands are thus the executive organs, or *effectors*, of the nervous system. We will deal with the structure of the effectors, as far as is necessary, in the relevant chapters.

Receptors. To react properly to its environment and to supervise the activity of the effectors, the nervous system also needs sensing elements that respond to changes in the environment and the organism and that transmit these responses to the nervous system. For this task the body possesses specialized nerve cells called *receptors*. We can therefore state that *specialized nerve cells that respond to certain changes in the organism or in its environment and that transmit these responses to the nervous system are called receptors.*

Each of these receptors responds to practically one particular form of stimulus only. The receptors of the eye, for example, react only to the stimulus of light or, more accurately, to electromagnetic radiation with a wavelength of 400 to 800 mμ (violet to red). These stimuli to which the receptors of the eye specifically react are called *adequate stimuli*. For most of the body's receptors we can say to which stimuli they are specially (specifically) sensitive, that is, we know their adequate stimuli. For example, sound waves (longitudinal fluctuations in air pressure) from 16 to 16,000 Hz (Hertz, cycles per second) constitute the adequate stimulus of the ear. High frequency sound waves are perceived as high-pitched sounds and low frequency waves as low-pitched sounds. (Receptors sometimes can also react to stimuli other than their adequate stimuli. However, in such cases, these *inadequate stimuli* must act on the receptor with a much greater amount of physical energy, for example, the "stars" that one sees when hit in the eye.)

It is through the receptors that the nervous system senses the events occurring in our environment and our bodies. In functional terms the receptors provide information on (1) our distant environment (eye, ear: teleceptors), (2) our immediate environment (skin receptors: exteroceptors), (3) the attitude and the position of the body in space (receptors of the muscles, the tendons, and the joints: proprioceptors), and (4) events in the intestines (interoceptors or visceroceptors).

The following questions will enable you to check your newly

acquired knowledge. When answering them you should avoid as far as possible checking back in the text.

Q 1.1 Which of the following statements are correct (one or more possibilities)? Note your answers on a sheet of paper and compare them with the answer key on page 277.
   a. Receptors react to all environmental stimuli.
   b. Each receptor has an adequate stimulus.
   c. Receptors are specialized nerve cells.
   d. The receptor is much more responsive to nonadequate (inadequate) than to adequate stimuli.
   e. Muscles and glands are the effectors of the nervous system.

Q 1.2 *Neuromuscular end plate* means the junction of an axon with a
   a. Smooth muscle fiber.
   b. Glandular cell.
   c. Skeletal muscle fiber.
   d. Nerve cell.
   e. Statements a to d are all incorrect.

Q 1.3 Draw a diagram of a neuron and label its various parts.

Q 1.4 Draw diagrams of and label the three typical junctions that are possible between two nerve cells.

Q 1.5 The cell bodies (somata) of the nerve cells range in diameter from
   a. 400 to 800 mμ.
   b. 5 to 100 μ.
   c. 0.1 to 1.0 mm.
   d. 16 to 16,000 Hz.
   e. they are more than 1 m in diameter.

1.2   Supporting and Alimentary Tissue

Glia cells.   While functionally the neurons are the most important building blocks of the nervous system, they are not the only cells of which the brain is composed. The neurons are encased in a special supporting tissue composed of *glia cells*, also known as neuroglia. In other organs of the body, this supporting tissue is generally referred to as connective tissue. Thus, the glia cells form the connective tissue of the nervous system. Besides their function as connective tissue, the glia cells are also thought to play a role in neuronal metabolism to some extent in certain processes of nervous excitation. However, there is considerable controversy surrounding these functions of the glia cells, and consequently these problems will not be examined in any further detail.

Extracellular space.   When examined under the light microscope the neurons and the glia cells look as if they abut each other in the nervous system without any interspace, like bricks laid without any mortar. Under the electron microscope, however, it is easy to see that a very narrow gap (average width: 200 Å = 20 mμ = 2 × 10^{-5} mm) separates the cells. All these interspaces are linked with one another to form the fluid-filled *extracellular space* of the neurons and the glia cells. At several points in the brain, known as the ventricles, the extracellular space widens to form large cavities. For more details, consult a book on neuroanatomy, examine anatomical specimen, or ask a butcher for an intact brain from a pig or calf which can then be cut into longitudinal and transverse sections to gain some idea of the arrangement of these cavities.

Because of its great functional importance, it must be stressed that there is no exchange of ions or nutrients directly between two neurons or a neuron and a glia cell. Such an exchange occurs always between the extracellular fluid and the neurons or glia cells. The fluid contained in the extracellular space is called *cerebrospinal fluid* or *liquor cerebrospinalis* (cerebrum = brain, spina = spine).

The extracellular space also surrounds the extremely thin branches of the blood vessels in the brain, the capillaries, and an exchange of material takes place between these and the extracellular space. Figure 1-5 shows diagrammatically the path of the oxygen (O_2) and the nutrients from the blood into the neuron and of the carbon dioxide (CO_2) and other metabolites from the neuron into the blood. A drug injected intravenously must therefore pass through the wall of the blood vessel (capillary membrane) and then through the cell membrane before it can take effect in a neuron. The capillary membrane of the cerebral

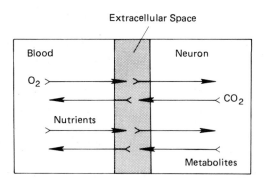

Fig. 1-5.   Neuronal supply pathways. The capillary blood vessel (*left*) and the neuron (*right*) are separated by the extracellular space. The arrows indicate the direction in which the nutrients and metabolites diffuse into and out of the extracellular space.

blood vessels seems to be impermeable to many substances, which is why pharmacologists speak of a "blood-brain barrier."

The neurons of the central nervous system, particularly those of the higher sections of the human brain (cerebral cortex), depend on a constant supply of oxygen. An interruption in the blood flow (for example, cardiac arrest, severe strangulation of the neck) for 8 to 12 sec is enough to cause unconsciousness. After 8 to 12 min irreversible brain damage usually has been sustained. When breathing stops, these times are considerably longer because the oxygen supply in the circulating blood can still be utilized.

Q 1.6 Which of the following statements is/are correct?
    a. Glia cells form the connective tissue of the nervous system.
    b. The fluid in the extracellular space and in the ventricle of the brain is called plasma.
    c. Complete lack of oxygen leads to irreversible brain damage only after several hours have elapsed.
    d. The extracellular space encloses all neurons but not the glia cells.
    e. The glia cells are filled with cerebrospinal fluid.
    f. None of the above statements is correct.

1.3 The Nerves

The *central nervous system* (CNS) consists of the *brain* and the *spinal cord*. All the remaining nervous tissue is referred to as the *peripheral nervous system*. The nerves in the periphery of the body are bundles of axons that are enclosed in their sheaths of connective tissue. Their structure, origin, and classification according to morphological and functional considerations will now be described.

The nerve fibers. A single axon is termed a *nerve fiber*. "Axon" and "nerve fiber" are thus synonyms, although the latter expression is more commonly used when referring to axons in the peripheral nerves. A *nerve* is a bundle of nerve fibers. If a nerve is big enough to be seen easily with the naked eye, it can contain as many as several hundred nerve fibers. In even thicker nerves the number of fibers can be tens of thousands. Upon emerging from the soma of the neuron, about 50 percent of all nerve fibers become encased in a sheath of lipoprotein (fat-protein mixture) called the *myelin*. In cross section such a nerve fiber resembles a wire encased in a thick insulating covering. Nerve fibers "insulated" in this way are called *myelinated* or *medullated nerve fibers*.

Unlike an insulated wire, the *medullary sheath* does not surround

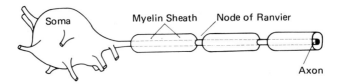

Fig. 1-6. Schematic three-dimensional diagram of a neuron with a medullated nerve fiber. The dendrites have been cut off. The medullary sheath, consisting of myelin, is interrupted at regular intervals by the nodes of Ranvier.

the nerve fiber continuously but, as illustrated in Fig. 1-6, is interrupted at regular intervals. Under the light microscope these unmedullated portions look like constrictions. They are therefore called the *nodes of Ranvier* after their discoverer. In myelinated nerve fibers a node of Ranvier occurs approximately every 1 to 2 mm. Nerve fibers without a medullary sheath are termed *unmedullated* or, since they are not covered by a myelin sheath, *unmyelinated nerve fibers.* Both types of nerve fibers, the medullated and the unmedullated, are enclosed in a sheath of special glia cells called *Schwann cells* after their discoverer. So, the axon is encased first in myelin, if it is myelinated, and then always in Schwann cells. Cross-sectional views through one myelinated and three unmyelinated nerve fibers and their associated Schwann cells are shown in Fig. 1-7. The Schwann cells surround the nerve fibers over their entire length, with each cell occupying approximately the space between two nodes. As Fig. 1-7 shows, in the case of the unmedullated nerve fibers a single Schwann cell often encloses several axons.

Physiologically, the medullated nerve fibers differ from the unmedullated fibers chiefly because of the different velocities at which both are capable of transmitting action potentials. For reasons explained in detail later, the conduction velocity is very high in myeli-

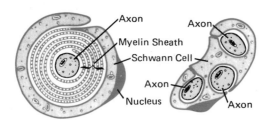

Fig. 1-7. Cross sections through medullated and unmedullated nerve fibers. The names of the two types of sheaths (myelin sheath, Schwann cells) are shown.

Table 1-1. Classification of Nerve Fibers.

Fiber Group			Diameter (μ)
Medullated fibers	I	⎫	18–10
(diam. = axon +	II	⎬ A fibers	10–5
medullary sheath)	III	⎭	5–1
Unmedullated fibers			
(diam. of axon)	IV	C fibers	1–0.1

nated nerve fibers and low in unmyelinated fibers. Within each group the conduction velocity also depends on the diameter of the axons: as the diameter increases the conduction velocity increases. Consequently, the various proposed anatomical and physiological classifications of nerve fibers coincide reasonably well. Medullated fibers are often referred to as *A fibers* and unmedullated fibers as *C fibers*. Table 1-1 shows the commonest classification according to diameter. The most frequently occurring diameters among the A fibers are those with values approximately equal to the mean values of the three ranges indicated, that is, 14, 7.5, and 3 μ.

Functional classification of nerve fibers. Apart from the conduction velocity and the diameter, a number of other functional characteristics are used to categorize nerve fibers. The most important of these are presented in Fig. 1-8. The nerve fibers of the receptors are called *afferent nerve fibers*, or, more succinctly, *afferents* (left side in Fig. 1-8). They lead to the CNS and transmit information from the receptors about changes in the environment or the body. Afferent nerve fibers from the intestines are termed *visceral afferents*, while all other afferents in the body—from muscles, joints, skin, and sensory organs of the head (eyes, ears, etc.)—are called *somatic* afferents.

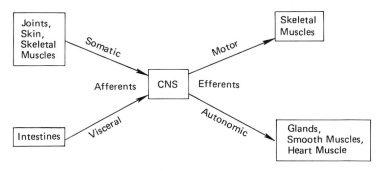

Fig. 1-8. Diagram of the classification of nerve fibers according to origin and function. See text for detailed discussion.

Transmission of information from the CNS to the periphery takes place by *efferent nerve fibers*, or, more succinctly, *efferents* (right side in Fig. 1-8). Efferents to the skeletal muscle fibers are called *motor* efferents. All the rest belong to the vegetative, or autonomic, nervous system and are therefore called *autonomic* efferents. The latter supply information to the smooth muscles of the intestines and in the walls of the blood vessels, as well as to the cardiac muscle and to all the glands in the body.

In the preceding paragraph we considered only the functional classification of individual nerve fibers. But, as we have already seen, a nerve contains large numbers, often many tens of thousands, of nerve fibers. In practically all nerves, for example, the Nervus ischiadicus, which innervates the greater part of the leg, afferent and efferent nerve fibers are bundled together. The types of nerve fiber contained in the nerve depend on the area (skin, muscles, intestines) it serves. It is now important to learn the names and the composition of these various nerves.

Classification of nerves. The nerves to the skin, the skeletal muscles, and the joints form the group known as *somatic* nerves. The nerves leading to the intestines are called *splanchnic nerves* (synonyms: autonomic nerves, visceral nerves, vegetative nerves; these terms are sometimes used with slightly different meanings, but we will not go into that here). A *cutaneous nerve* is thus a somatic nerve. It contains somatic afferents (afferent nerve fibers) from the receptors of the skin, but it also contains autonomic efferents to the blood vessels, the sweat glands, and the skin hair. A skeletal muscle nerve, usually called a *muscle nerve* for short, is also a somatic nerve. It contains motor efferents as well as somatic afferents from the receptors of the muscles and autonomic efferents to the blood vessels. A *joint nerve* is also a somatic nerve with somatic afferents from the receptors of the joints and autonomic efferents to the blood vessels of the joints and the joint capsule. The thick nerves, for example, Nervus ischiadicus, are usually *mixed nerves* that later branch into their component cutaneous, muscle, and joint nerves. Finally, we must mention that the *splanchnic nerves* contain visceral afferents and autonomic efferents.

You should now be able to give the correct answers to the following questions:

Q 1.7 Which of the following statements is/are correct?
a. Cutaneous, muscle, and splanchnic nerves form a group known as somatic nerves.
b. Unmedullated fibers are always larger in diameter than the medullated type.

    c. "Somatic afferents" and "somatic nerves" are synonymous terms.

    d. A cutaneous nerve has no motor efferents.

Q 1.8 By "nodes of Ranvier," we mean

    a. The points where an axon branches into its collaterals.

    b. The indentations in the Schwann cells caused by the unmedullated nerve fibers embedded in them.

    c. The regular interruptions in the medullary sheath in the case of myelinated nerve fibers.

    d. The gaps, filled with cerebrospinal fluid, between the cells of the CNS.

    e. The point of transition of the receptor into the afferent nerve fiber.

Q 1.9 The diameter of medullated nerve fibers is in the order of magnitude of

    a. 0.1–1 μ d. 0.1–1.0 mm

    b. 1–20 μ e. 1–10 mm

    c. 20–100 μ

1.4 The Anatomy of the Central Nervous System (CNS)

Of the two parts of the CNS, the brain and the spinal cord, the latter is phylogenetically by far the older and is relatively simple and stereotyped in structure. We will now study the structure of the spinal cord and, at the same time, gain an initial impression of the arrangement of the neurons in the CNS.

The structure of a spinal segment. The brain and the spinal cord are enclosed in bony protective casings (Fig. 1-9), the *skull* and the *vertebral canal*, respectively. As a result of this design the soft tissue of the CNS is optimally protected from mechanical damage. One section of the spinal cord, a *spinal segment*, corresponds to each vertebra. This uniform structure has been determined by evolutionary factors. As a person grows, however, the growth of the spinal segments falls behind that of the vertebrae so that, as the longitudinal (sagittal) section in Fig. 1-9 shows, in adult humans the spinal cord ends at approximately the level of the top lumbar vertebrae, although the segmented structure is fully retained.

The uniform structure of the spinal cord in the longitudinal direction, that is, the way it is built up of spinal segments, is matched by a uniform cross-sectional structure in all parts. Figure 1-10 illustrates such a cross section. The cell bodies of the neurons are located in the inner region of the spinal cord, and the ascending and the descending

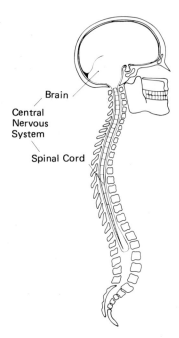

Fig. 1-9. Diagrammatic longitudinal section through the center line (sagittal section) of skull and spinal column. The boundaries of the segments in the spinal cord are drawn to show the relationship with the vertebrae.

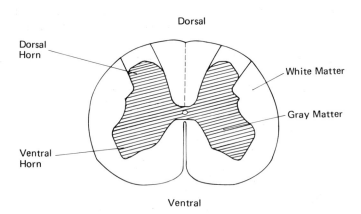

Fig. 1-10. Cross section through the spinal cord at the level of a lumbar segment. In other sections of the spinal cord the shape of the gray matter and the ratio of the gray to the white matter are slightly different from what is shown here. (See text.)

nerve fibers are located in the outer regions. In fresh section, the cell bodies (unstained and viewed with the naked eye) appear gray in color. Therefore this region of the spinal cord, which is butterfly-shaped in cross section, is called the *gray matter*. The anterior (ventral) part of each butterfly wing is called the *ventral horn*, the side (lateral) part is called the *lateral horn*, and the posterior (dorsal) part the *dorsal horn*. The part of the gray matter located medially (toward the center) from the lateral horn is called the *pars intermedia*.

The butterfly-shaped gray matter, which forms the portion of a spinal segment, is encased by the ascending and the descending nerve fibers, which form the outer regions of the segment. The myelin makes the nerve fibers appear white in cross section; therefore these regions are referred to as the *white matter*. The ratio of white to gray matter is not the same in all sections of the spinal cord. In the cervical and the thoracic segments, which are located closer to the brain, the proportion of white matter in the overall cross section is particularly large because all the ascending and the descending pathways pass through these segments, while only the pathways from the lower regions of the body run in the lumbar and the sacral segments.

Spinal cord roots.   In each spinal segment, nerve fibers enter the spinal cord at the dorsal (posterior) side and emerge from the spinal cord at the ventral (anterior) side. Figure 1-11 is a cross section through such a zone with *dorsal* and *ventral* roots. All the afferent fibers, the somatic as well as the visceral afferents, thus enter the spinal cord in the dorsal roots. All efferent nerve fibers, that is, the motor and the autonomic efferents, emerge from the spinal cord in the ventral roots only.

The cell bodies of the efferent fibers are located in the gray matter

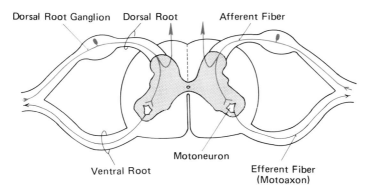

Fig. 1-11.   Diagrammatic cross section through the spinal cord at the level of a root entry zone.

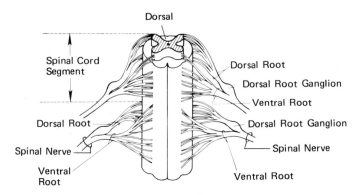

Fig. 1-12. Three-dimensional representation of two spinal cord segments with their roots. See text for details.

of the spinal cord. The cell bodies of the motor efferent fibers, which lead to the skeletal muscle fibers, are situated in the ventral horn. Because of their position, these cells therefore are called *ventral horn cells*, and because of their function they are called *motor* ventral horn cells, or *motoneurons*. Their axons, that is, the motor nerve fibers, are also often called motoaxons. (A description of the position of the somata of the autonomic efferents is given in Chapter 9.)

In contrast to the efferent fibers, whose cell bodies are located in the gray matter of the spinal cord, the cell bodies of all the afferent fibers are situated outside the spinal cord and close to where the roots enter the vertebral canal. Such a local accumulation of nerve cells outside the CNS is called a *ganglion*. The accumulation of the cell bodies of the dorsal root afferents is called a *dorsal root ganglion*. The neurons in the dorsal root ganglion have three special characteristics: their axons divide shortly after emerging into the centrally projecting (dorsal root fibers) and the peripherally projecting (afferent fibers) branches, the soma has no dendrites, and there are no synapses on the soma. Figure 1-3d shows a dorsal root ganglion cell.

These structures are summarized and further clarified by the three-dimensional drawing of two spinal segments and their roots in Fig. 1-12. While still in the vertebral canal, the individual ventral and dorsal root filaments of each spinal half-segment come together to form common ventral and dorsal roots, respectively. In the dorsal root, the spinal ganglion appears as a distinct thickening. On both sides of the cord, the ventral and the dorsal root join to form the spinal nerve, which then emerges from the vertebral canal at an appropriate gap between two vertebrae. Only after the spinal nerves emerge from the vertebral canal do their various somatic and autonomic nerve components separate from each other through a complex process of interlacing and branching. The nerves emerging from the spinal cord serve the entire body, with the exception of the head, which is served by 12 paired cranial nerves. Relevant details and special information will be given later in the text.

The anatomy presented in this chapter is sufficient to understand Chapters 2 to 4. In the later chapters, any new anatomical information will be introduced when needed. The following questions will help you check whether you have mastered the material presented in this chapter.

Q 1.10 Draw a diagram of a nerve cell and label the various parts of this cell. Draw a diagram of, and label the possible connections between, two nerve cells.

Q 1.11 The cells of the brain are separated from each other and from the blood capillaries by a narrow gap. What is this gap called? What is the name of the fluid it contains?

Q 1.12 What types of afferent and efferent nerve fibers are contained in the N. ischiadicus of human beings?

Q 1.13 Which of the following statements is/are correct?
   a. Each spinal segment has two ventral roots.
   b. One half of a spinal segment corresponds to each vertebra.
   c. The motoneurons are located in the dorsal root ganglia.
   d. The gray matter of the spinal cord owes its coloration to the myelin sheaths.
   e. The cell bodies of the dorsal root ganglia cells have no synapses.
   f. Each spinal segment has one dorsal root.

Q 1.14 Which of the following descriptions of nerve fibers contains mutually exclusive or contradictory concepts?
   a. Myelinated, afferent, soma in ventral horn.
   b. Unmyelinated, afferent, diameter 10 μ.
   c. In mixed nerve, efferent, motoneuron.
   d. Visceral, efferent, soma in dorsal root ganglion.
   e. Afferent, visceral, unmyelinated, efferent.

2

EXCITATION OF NERVE
AND MUSCLE

A difference in potential, the *membrane potential*, usually exists between the inside of a cell and the extracellular fluid surrounding it. In many types of cells, for example, muscle cells or glandular cells, the function of the cell can be controlled by the magnitude of this potential. It is, in fact, the specialized role of the nervous system to propagate changes in membrane potential within its cells and to transmit them to other cells. These changes in potential can be regarded as units of information that help the body to coordinate the activity of various groups of cells. In particular, the body can feed the information impinging on it from the environment to a center where it is processed, enabling the body to adapt itself in a suitable manner to its surroundings. At the basis of all these functions is the membrane potential and the changes in this potential that spread out through the cells. How the membrane potential is generated and what conditions govern its changes will be discussed in detail in this chapter.

2.1   Resting Potential

Measuring the membrane potential.   The potential difference between the interior of a cell and the fluid surrounding the cell—the *membrane potential*—can be measured by connecting one pole of a voltmeter to the inside of the cell and the other pole to the extracellular space. The appropriate apparatus is diagrammed in Fig. 2-1A. The voltmeter is connected through the electrodes to the test preparation, a cell which is maintained in a bath solution. Usually glass capillaries filled with a conducting solution are used as the electrodes, which can be inserted into the interior of the cell. In order not to damage the cells, these glass capillaries have very fine tips (less than $1\ \mu$). At the

16

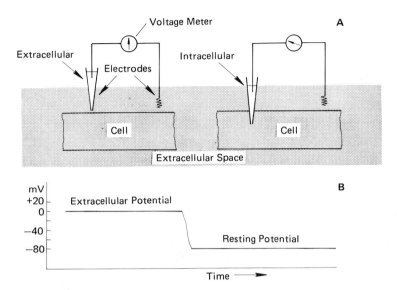

Fig. 2-1. Measuring the intracellular membrane potential. *A*: Diagram of the measuring setup. The cell is located in an extracellular space filled with a blood substitute solution. In the left-hand diagram the reference electrode and the recording electrode are both outside the cell and the voltage meter connected between them shows zero potential. In the right-hand diagram the recording electrode has been inserted into the cell while the reference electrode remains in its extracellular location. The voltage meter now records the membrane potential. *B*: The membrane potential recorded before and after insertion of the recording electrode.

start of the measurement (left half of Fig. 2-1*A*) both electrodes are located in the extracellular space, and no potential difference exists between them. The potential of the extracellular space is generally agreed to be 0. This zero potential is indicated in Fig. 2-1*B* (left) as the "extracellular potential." When the tip of the glass capillary is pushed through the membrane of the cell (Fig. 2-1*A*, right), the potential jumps in a negative direction to approximately − 75 mV, as is shown in Fig. 2-1*B*. Since this potential difference occurs when the membrane is penetrated, it is referred to as the *membrane potential*.

In most cells, the membrane potential remains constant for a fairly long time, provided that no special influences act on the cell from the outside. When the cell is in such a resting state, the membrane potential is called the *resting potential*. The resting potential is always negative in nerve and muscle cells and has a characteristic constant magnitude for the individual cell types. In the nerve and the skeletal muscle fibers of warm-blooded animals, the resting potentials are between −55 and −100 mV. In smooth muscle fibers more positive resting potentials between −55 and −30 mV occur.

Origin of the resting potential. What physical processes generate the resting potential? If the interior of the cell has a greater negative charge than the surroundings of the cell, then excess negative electric charges will exist within the cell compared with that of the extracellular space. Both the inside of the cell and the extracellular space are filled with aqueous salt solutions. In dilute salt solutions the majority of the molecules dissociate into ions, that is, positively or negatively charged atoms or groups of atoms. Positively charged atoms or molecules are called *cations*; negatively charged ones are called *anions* (because in an electrical field they migrate to the cathode or the anode, respectively). When, for example, sodium chloride (NaCl) is dissolved in water it dissociates into the cation Na^+ and the anion Cl^-. In aqueous solutions the ions are the sole carriers of charge. Consequently, charge disequilibrium, which is expressed by the resting potential, indicates a certain excess of anions (negative charges) inside the cell and a corresponding excess of cations outside the cell.

Since ions can move freely in an aqueous solution, a disequilibrium in charge cannot continue to exist within either the intracellular or the extracellular space; it must be balanced out by the movement of the ions. The charge disequilibrium which causes the resting potential therefore must be located at the "solid phase" which demarcates the cell, that is, the cell membrane. The resting potential is thus generated at the cell membrane; on the inner side, within the cell, there is an excess of anions, while on the outer side there is a corresponding excess of cations.

The *cell membrane* can be regarded as an *electric capacitor* in which two conducting media, the intracellular and the extracellular salt solutions, are separated from one another by a nonconducting layer, the membrane. The insulating membrane is about 6 mμ (60 Å) thick. In order to charge a capacitor with this "plate spacing" to the resting potential of −75 mV, it must carry approximately 5,000 pairs of ions per square micron of cell surface. The electric potential at the capacitor is proportional to the number of charges that are held on its "plates."

In order to clarify further the numerical ratios of the ions involved, Fig. 2-2 shows a very small section of the membrane measuring 1 μ × 1/1000 μ in area and the adjoining intra- and extracellular volumes, each 1 μ 1 μ × 1/1000 μ. Assuming a resting potential of –90mV, this membrane area is occupied by six anions and six cations. However, there are 220,000 ions in each of the adjoining spaces. The imbalance

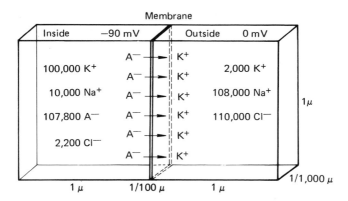

Fig. 2-2. Membrane charge during resting potential. The charge of a small section of the membrane measuring $1\ \mu \times 1/1000\ \mu$ in area with six K^+ ions and six anions is contrasted with the number of ions in adjacent spaces, each $1\ \mu \times 1\ \mu \times 1/1000\ \mu$, on either side of the membrane. A^- denotes the intracellular protein anions. The arrows through the membrane indicate that the K^+ has diffused through the membrane from the cell but remains fixed to the outside of the membrane because of the charge of the A^- remaining in the cell.

in the distribution of the charge at the membrane is very slight, nevertheless it is the basis of the resting potential and thus of the functioning of the nervous system.

Distribution of the ion concentrations.   Why is it always a negative resting potential that occurs in nerve and muscle? The source of the resting potential is the *unequal distribution of the types of ions*, particularly the K^+ ions, inside and outside the cell. The distribution of the various types of ions for the intracellular and the extracellular spaces is given in Fig. 2-2. The largest disequilibrium exists in the case of the K^+ ions: these number 100,000 on the intracellular side and only 2,000 on the extracellular side. The figures for Na^+, on the other hand, are 108,000 outside and only 10,000 inside the cell. The distribution of the Cl^- ions is exactly the reverse of the K^+ ions. The majority of the intracellular anions are not chloride but large protein anions, designated as A^-.

Table 2-1 gives the *ionic concentrations inside* and *outside* the *muscle cell* of a mammal (in mM). In these cells the potassium concentration in the cell is about 40 times higher than in the extracellular space, and the sodium concentration is about 12 times higher outside than inside. These ionic distributions are very constant in the individual types of cell. Generally, in nerve and muscle cells the intracellular K^+ concentration is 20 to 100 times greater than the extracellular

Table 2-1.   Ionic Concentrations Inside and Outside
the Muscle Cell of a Mammal (mM).

Intracellular		Extracellular	
Na⁺	12	Na⁺	145
K⁺	155	K⁺	4
		Other cations	4
Cl⁻	4	Cl⁻	120
HCO₃⁻	8	HCO₃⁻	27
A⁻	155		
Resting potential: -90 mV			

concentration, the intracellular Na⁺ concentration is 5 to 15 times lower than the extracellular concentration, and the intracellular Cl⁻ concentration is 20 to 100 times lower than the extracellular figure. The concentration distribution of chloride is thus approximately reciprocal to that of K⁺. The extracellular salt solution is essentially a sodium chloride solution with an NaCl content of about 9 g/liter. A solution of 9 g of sodium chloride in 1 liter of water is also called a *"physiological saline solution."* This solution tastes just as salty as blood.

The K⁺ ions and the resting potential.   How is the resting potential generated by the different ionic concentrations in the extracellular and the intracellular spaces? The different ionic concentrations would soon cancel each other by *diffusion* of the mobile particles if this were not prevented by the cell membrane. If the membrane constituted an impenetrable barrier for ions, that is, if it were *impermeable*, the different ionic concentrations on both sides of the membrane could continue to exist without restriction. However, the membrane is not completely impermeable but permits K⁺ ions to pass through with relative ease. In other words, it is *permeable to K⁺ ions*. We can therefore picture the membrane as being full of pores or canals as indicated in Fig. 2-3. These pores are so narrow that only the relatively small K⁺ ions can traverse them, diffusing through the membrane. The "size" of the ions in Fig. 2-3 corresponds to their effective diameter. This is not the same as the "ion radius": in aqueous solution water molecules become attached to the ions, and the latter become hydrated. The hydrated K⁺ ions are smaller than the hydrated Na⁺ ions; see this relationship in Fig. 2-3.

In order to represent the *diffusion conditions* at the membrane, all the ions except the K⁺ ions have been omitted from Fig. 2-4 because it is only the K⁺ that can pass through the membrane. The K⁺ ions will move through the membrane in both directions, that is, from outside

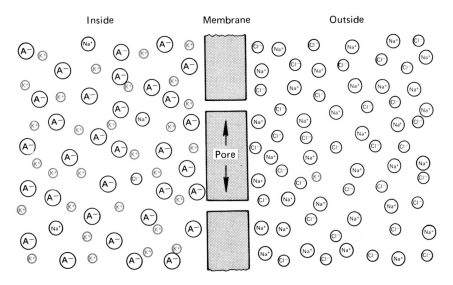

Fig. 2-3. Intra- and extracellular distribution of the ions. On both sides of the membrane the different ions are indicated by different size circles. The diameter is in each case proportional to the (hydrated) ion diameter. A⁻ designates the large intracellular protein anions. The passages through the membrane, the "pores," are just large enough to permit the K⁺ ions to diffuse through.

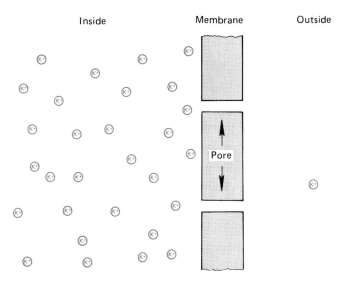

Fig. 2-4. Intra- and extracellular distribution of K⁺ ions. This is the same diagram as Fig. 2-3, but all ions, with the exception of K⁺, have been omitted, since only the latter can pass through the membrane.

to inside and vice versa. But because of their higher concentration within the cell, the K⁺ ions will find and pass through a pore on the inner side approximately 30 times more frequently than on the outer side. A net efflux of K⁺ ions results, the motive force being the higher *osmotic pressure of K⁺* inside the cell. The osmotic pressure difference for K⁺ would very soon lead to an equalization of the K⁺ concentrations as a result of the K⁺ efflux were it not for an equally large and opposite-acting force preventing this.

The opposing force is supplied by an electric field, the *membrane potential*, the origin of which will now be explained. We have so far ignored the fact that the K⁺ ions carry *positive charges*. As was discussed in connection with Fig. 2-2, the shifting of a cation across the cell membrane results in the *membrane capacitor becoming charged* and gives rise to a membrane potential. When a K⁺ ion flows out of the cell an excess positive charge will appear on the outer side of the capacitor, corresponding to an excess negative charge on the inner side. The membrane potential acts in such a way that it opposes the efflux of more cations. The efflux of positive charges by itself builds up an electric potential that impedes the efflux of more positive charges. The electric potential builds up until the force that it exerts against the efflux of K⁺ ions is equal to the osmotic pressure of the K⁺ ions. At this potential the influx and the efflux of K⁺ ions are balanced, and we therefore refer to it as the *K⁺ equilibrium potential, or E_K.*

The potassium equilibrium potential, E_K, is determined by the concentration ratio of the K⁺ ions inside and outside the cell, K^+_i/K^+_o. E_K is proportional to the logarithm of this concentration ratio. The quantitative relationship between concentration ratio and equilibrium potential is called the *Nernst equation*. For K⁺ ions this equation reads:

$$E_K = -61 \text{ mV} \cdot \log (K^+_i/K^+_o)$$

The factor −61 mV is derived from a series of constants and the temperature.* If $K^+_i/K^+_o = 30$, as in Fig. 2-3 and 2-4, then

$$E_K = -61 \text{ mV} \cdot \log 30 = -61 \text{ mV} \cdot 1.48 = -90 \text{ mV}$$

that is, it is approximately as large as the resting potential. The *resting potential*, as a first approximation, thus corresponds to the *potassium*

---

*In general form the Nernst equation is written as follows:

$$E_{ion} = \frac{R \cdot T}{z \cdot F} \cdot \ln \frac{\text{Extracellular ionic concentration}}{\text{Intracellular ionic concentration}}$$

in which R is the gas constant, F the Faraday constant, z the valence of the ion (positive for cations and negative for anions), and T the absolute temperature.

equilibrium potential. At this potential the concentration difference of the K^+ ions across the membrane can remain unchanged, despite the good permeability for K^+, because the membrane potential is just large enough to prevent a net efflux of K^+.

Role of Cl^- in the resting potential. The representation of the resting potential as a potassium equilibrium potential must be amended to take account of the fact that the chloride ions are also involved. The *membranes* are in fact also *permeable for Cl^- ions.* In nerve cells the permeability to Cl^- is less than to K^+, but in muscle cells it is much greater than that to K^+. The concentration ratio of chloride ions inside and outside the cell, Cl^-_i/Cl^-_o, is usually reciprocal to the corresponding concentration ratio K^+_i/K^+_o (see Table 2-1). For this reciprocal distribution of the chloride, we find, in accordance with the Nernst equation (for anions the sign is reversed), the same potential as for the potassium distribution. The *chloride equilibrium potential* is, then, approximately equal to the *potassium equilibrium potential.*

The reciprocal distribution of K^+ and Cl^- across the cell membrane does not happen by chance. The intracellular chloride concentration can be varied easily by the influx or the efflux of Cl^-, and adjusts itself according to the membrane potential, because when the chloride equilibrium potential deviates from the membrane potential, compensatory currents flow. If the membrane potential adjusts itself at E_K the result is a Cl^- distribution reciprocal to the K^+ distribution and E_{Cl} becomes equal to E_K.

Unlike the Cl^- concentration, the intracellular K^+ concentration cannot change very much. The K^+ ions must in fact provide the charge in the cell to balance out the anions. The intracellular anions are mainly large protein molecules (see Table 2-1), which cannot pass through the cell membrane, so their concentration remains constant. These large anions must be opposed in the intracellular solution by an equal number of cations. Since the intracellular Na^+ concentration is kept very low (see Sec. 2-3), neutrality of charge must be guaranteed by K^+ ions. It follows, therefore, that the intracellular K^+ concentration must be about as high as that of the large anions and that the intracellular K^+ concentration, just as that of the large anions, must be very stable. The high intracellular concentration of $\overset{.}{K}^+$ is indirectly necessitated by the presence of the nonpermeable intracellular anions, and, in turn, the negative E_K derives from this high intracellular concentration of K^+. The Cl^- concentration in the cell depends on the membrane potential and is a secondary result of the K^+ distribution. From this standpoint, the negative resting potential is the result of the high concentration of nonpermeable anions in the cell.

The following questions are intended to check what you have learned so far.

Q 2.1 Draw a diagram of the test apparatus used for the intracellular measurement of the membrane potential of a cell. At the same time, show at the membrane of the cell the charge of the membrane potential with the cations and the anions that are essential for the resting potential.

Q 2.2 Enter in the following table the ratio of the intracellular to the extracellular ion concentration for K^+, Na^+, and Cl^- ions.

Ion	Internal/External	
K^+	_____-_____ /	1
Na^+	1	/ _____-_____
Cl^-	1	/ _____-_____

The distribution of K^+ and Cl^- ions is _____.

Q 2.3 Which of the following variables are in balance at the equilibrium potential for an ion?
  a. The intracellular and the extracellular concentrations of the ion.
  b. Osmotic pressure and electric field.
  c. Influx and efflux of the ion through the cell membrane.
  d. The Na^+ concentration outside the cell and the K^+ concentration inside the cell.

2.2   Resting Potential and Na^+ Influx

The explanation of the resting potential given in the preceding section—that it is determined by the K^+ equilibrium potential—proceeded from the simplifying assumption that the cell membrane is permeable only to K^+ and Cl^- ions. By making this assumption it was possible to demonstrate a diffusion and potential equilibrium across the cell membrane. However, to a lesser extent the membrane is also permeable to Na^+ and other ions. Flows of these ions disturb the equilibrium so that a constant resting potential cannot be maintained by diffusion processes alone.

Dependence of the resting potential on the potassium concentration.   The statement that the *resting potential* is the same as the *potassium equilibrium potential* can be checked experimentally. The extracellular K^+ concentration can be varied within wide limits, and at the same time the resting potential can be measured. Such resting potentials, measured for various extracellular K^+ concentrations, K^+_o, are plotted as circles in Fig. 2-6. When the extracellular K^+ concentra-

Fig. 2-5 appears on page 277 as an answer to Q. 2.1.

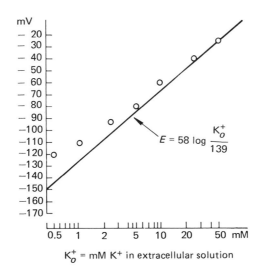

$$E = 58 \log \frac{K_o^+}{139}$$

K_o^+ = mM K^+ in extracellular solution

Fig. 2-6. Dependence of the resting potential on the extracellular K^+ concentration. The abscissa shows the extracellular K_o^+ plotted on a logarithmic scale; the ordinate gives the membrane potential. The circles correspond to the membrane potentials measured at various values of K^+. The straight line is that of the potassium equilibrium potentials as determined by the Nernst equation at various values of K_o^+. (From Adrian, *J. Physiol.* **133,** 631, 1956.)

tion is increased, the resting potential decreases from -90 to -20 mV. In addition, E_K can be calculated in accordance with the Nernst equation for the various extracellular K^+ concentrations. This calculated dependence of E_K on K^+_o is shown as a straight line in Fig. 2-6. The relationship is linear because K^+_o is plotted on a logarithmic scale along the abscissa. The measurements agree essentially with the calculated straight line and, to a first approximation, confirm the proposal that the resting potential is the same as the potassium equilibrium potential. It will be noticed, however, that only in the upper region of the curve, that is, at high K^+_o values, do the measurements agree well with the theoretical relationship, while at low K^+_o values they deviate upward to an increasing extent. Thus, at low extracellular K^+ concentrations the resting potential is less negative than E_K. This is also true for the normal extracellular K^+ concentration of about 4 mM. In muscle fibers, as illustrated here, as well as in other types of cell, the *resting potential is up to 30 mV less negative than the E_K.*

An indication of why the resting potential deviates from E_K at low extracellular K^+ concentrations can be obtained from a variation of the experiment illustrated in Fig. 2-6. If the same experiment is carried out in a bathing solution in which the Na^+ is replaced by a large cation that cannot pass through the membrane (for example, choline), then the measured resting potential and the calculated E_K agree exactly even at low K^+. The deviation of the resting potential from E_K in a Na^+-containing solution must therefore be caused by a flow of Na^+ ions through the cell membrane. It can be concluded that in the resting condition, the membrane is permeable to not only K^+ ions but also, to a lesser extent, Na^+ ions. As a result, the Na^+ ions, which are present in very much higher concentrations on the outside, flow slowly into the cell, partly discharge the membrane capacitor, and make the membrane potential less negative.

Membrane conductance for K^+ and Na^+. The resting potential usually does not quite agree with E_K because the membrane is permeable to not only potassium (and chloride ions) but also to some extent *sodium ions*. The degree to which the resting potential deviates from E_K is determined by the ratio of the membrane permeability values for Na^+ and K^+. In order to give a quantitative explanation of the resting potential it is therefore necessary in some way to measure the ionic permeability of the membrane. For this purpose it is usually the *membrane conductance, g*, which is determined. The conductance is the reciprocal of the electric resistance. The electric resistance is determined by the quotient of voltage/current; consequently, the conductance is determined as g = current/voltage. To obtain the membrane conductance for a certain ion the flux through the membrane of the ions in question must be divided by the potential that provides the driving force. This driving potential is 0 at the equilibrium potential because at this latter potential the net ion flux is equal to zero. The equilibrium potential should be taken as the reference point for the driving potential. As the membrane potential moves further away from the equilibrium potential, the influx and efflux become more and more out of balance, and the net flow increases. Therefore, the distance between the membrane potential and the equilibrium potential is taken as the driving potential for the (net) ionic flux. We can then write for the *potassium conductance*

$$g_K = I_K/(E\text{-}E_K)$$

in which I_K is the net potassium flux and E is the membrane potential. Experimental quantitative determinations of g_K and g_{Na} have shown that under resting conditions in nerve and muscle cells g_K is *10 to 25 times larger than* g_{Na}.

From the equilibrium potential and the conductances for K^+ and Na^+ ions it is now possible to explain the magnitude of the resting potential for various K^+_o values. The *sodium equilibrium potential*

E_{Na} is situated at positive potentials because the Na^+ concentration inside the cell is smaller than outside. The quotient Na^+_i/Na^+_o is smaller than 1, and thus log Na^+_i/Na^+_o is negative. When the ratio Na^+_i to Na^+_o = 1:12, we obtain, according to the Nernst equation (see page 22).

$$E_{Na} = -61 \text{ mV} \cdot \log 1/12 = -61 \text{ mV} \cdot (-1.08) = +65 \text{ mV}$$

If the potential is more negative than E_{Na} a net sodium current enters the cell. This, in fact, obtains over the entire potential range in Fig. 2-6. If g_{Na} remains constant in this potential range, then the sodium inward current becomes greater as the deviation from E_{Na} increases $\left[I_{Na} = g_{Na} \cdot (E\text{-}E_{Na})\right]$. Thus, as the membrane potential becomes more negative in Fig. 2-6, the Na^+ inward current increases, causing a larger deviation of the resting potential from E_K.

Even at the normal extracellular K^+ concentration the resting potential is about 10 mV less negative than E_K. This can be explained quantitatively by the ratio of g_K to g_{Na} and by the deviations of the resting potential from E_K and E_{Na}. At the resting potential a small potassium outward current must be in equilibrium with an sodium inward current. If these currents are to be equal, the 20 times greater conductance for K^+ must be offset by a 20 times greater driving potential for Na^+. The following relationships must exist:

$$g_K : g_{Na} = 20 : 1$$
$$-(E - E_{Na}) : (E - E_K) = 20 : 1$$

From the latter expression it follows that

$$E = E_K + \frac{E_{Na} - E_K}{21}$$

$E_{Na} - E_K = +65 - (-90)$ mV = 155 mV; according to this calculation the resting potential E would be 7.4 mV more positive than E_K.

Instability of the resting potential given purely passive ionic currents. The fact that under resting conditions Na^+ ions continuously flow into the cells, while, correspondingly, K^+ ions must flow out, has far-reaching consequences. The system cannot, in fact, be equilibrated under resting conditions by means of diffusion and buildup of membrane charge alone; this would mean that the intracellular ionic concentrations could not be kept constant. If no other processes (see Sec. 2.3) were involved besides the *passive* ion currents mentioned above, the cell would slowly pick up more Na^+ and lose K^+. The decline in intracellular K^+ concentration would bring about a decrease in E_K and thus in the resting potential. As their resting potential declined to less negative values the intracellular Cl⁻ concentration would be forced to rise because it adjusts itself to the resting potential. The large intracellular protein anions cannot leave the cell, so as the intracellular Cl⁻ concentration rose, there would be an increase in the total intracellular anion concentration and consequently in the total ion concentration. In order to equalize the osmotic pressure, water would flow into the cell, and the cell volume would expand. In turn, the water picked up by the cell would lower the intracellular K⁺ concentration and so reduce the membrane potential. Thus, with the takeup of water and the decline in the resting potential, the intracellular ion concentrations would nearly match the extracellular concentrations.

The process that prevents all this from happening in healthy, living cells is discussed in the next section.

Now check the knowledge you have acquired in this section.

Q 2.4 Which of the following statements indicate that, apart from K^+ and Cl^- ions, Na^+ ions also influence the resting potential?
   a. The resting potential is less negative than E_K.
   b. The resting potential changes approximately in proportion to the logarithm of the extracellular K^+ concentration.
   c. In the absence of extracellular Na^+ the resting potential and E_K are the same.
   d. The sodium equilibrium potential is positive while the potassium equilibrium potential is negative.

Q 2.5 What is the equation used to define the chloride conductance of the membrane?

Q 2.6 Where would the membrane potential be if the membrane were permeable only to Na^+? Give the symbol and the approximate value for this potential.

Q 2.7 Which of the following statements show why the resting membrane potential is made more positive by the inflow of Na^+?
   a. There are more Na^+ ions outside the cell than inside.
   b. The cell loses K^+ ions because of the inflow of Na^+ ions.
   c. The negative charge on the inner side of the membrane is reduced by the influx of Na^+ ions.
   d. The cell also picks up chloride as a result of the Na^+ inflow.

2.3 The Sodium Pump

The preceding section showed how the diffusion of Na^+ ions into the cell during resting conditions could upset the equilibrium of the ionic currents to such an extent that the normal concentration gradients and the resting potential would slowly disappear. The Na^+ ions flowing *passively* into the cell must leave the cell again; otherwise the intracellular Na^+ concentration could not remain at a constant low level. The Na^+ ions that have entered the cell cannot leave again by diffusion against the potential and the concentration gradients, that is, they cannot flow "uphill."* They must therefore be expelled *actively* from the cell, which requires the expenditure of energy. The passive inflow of Na^+ is in fact balanced by *active transport* of Na^+ from the cell. This transport mechanism is also called the *sodium pump*. The sodium pump transports Na^+ ions from the cell against the concentration and the potential gradients with the expenditure of metabolic energy.

Measuring the active transport of Na^+. The active transport of Na^+ ions out of the cell can be determined by measuring the Na^+ efflux from the cell. The number of Na^+ ions that can leave the cell passively against the concentration and the potential gradients is negligibly small. The Na^+ efflux from the cell is thus identical to the number of ions actively transported. In order to measure the Na^+ ions that have flowed out of the cell, it is necessary to distinguish them from the many other Na^+ ions already present in the extracellular space. This can be done by first loading the cell intracellularly with a *radioactive isotope of sodium* ($^{24}Na^+$) and then measuring the occurrence of this isotope in the extracellular space.

Figure 2-7 illustrates two such experiments conducted on a nerve. In part *A* during the first measurement period at 18.3°C, the $^{24}Na^+$ efflux slowly declines, because, as a result of the efflux itself, the $^{24}Na^+$ fraction of the intracellular Na^+ concentration drops. If the *temperature of the nerve* is suddenly *lowered* to 0.5°C, the $^{24}Na^+$ *efflux immediately drops* to about one-tenth its value. When the temperature of the nerve is increased again, the rate of $^{24}Na^+$ efflux returns to the value observed prior to cooling. The strong dependence of the Na^+ efflux on temperature shows that an *active chemical process,* and not passive diffusion, is involved. Diffusion processes would be slowed down only slightly by a drop in temperature. Therefore, active transport must be involved in the Na^+ efflux.

Further proof is provided by a variation of the experiment on which Fig. 2-7*B* is based. At the start of the experiment, $^{24}Na^+$ flows out of the cell at a fast rate. When dinitrophenol (DNP) is added to the extracellular solution, the $^{24}Na^+$ efflux drops to almost zero within an hour. After the DNP is flushed out, the normal $^{24}Na^+$ efflux picks up again. DNP is a poison that penetrates the cell and blocks energy-

---

*Of course, these statements only apply to a net sodium efflux. A very small fraction of the intracellular Na^+, compared with the rate of influx, can diffuse outward.

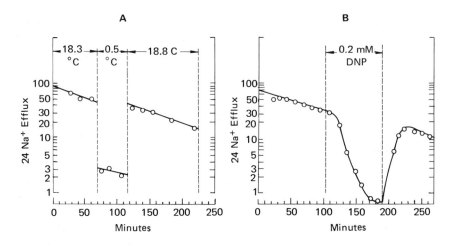

Fig. 2-7. Inhibition of active Na^+ transport as a result of cooling or exposure to dinitrophenol (DNP). Efflux of radioactive $^{24}Na^+$ from a cell into which this isotope was loaded before the start of the experiment. Abscissa: Time after start of experiment in minutes. Ordinate: Efflux of $^{24}Na^+$ from the cell. A: During the experiment the cell is cooled from 18.3°C to 0.5°C and warmed again. The Na^+ efflux is severely reduced during the cold period. B: During the experiment the cell is exposed for 90 min to 0.2 mM dinitrophenol, thereby causing a drop in the Na^+ efflux to almost 0. After the DNP has been flushed out the efflux starts up again. (From Hodgkin and Keynes: *J. Physiol.* **128**, 28, 1955.)

supplying metabolic processes. Diffusion processes through the membrane are not affected by DNP. The drop in the Na^+ efflux in the presence of DNP is due to an inadequate supply of metabolic energy. This demonstrates that the *Na^+ efflux is dependent on the availability of energy* and therefore that Na^+ is actively transported through the membrane.

Even in the living organism the supply of adequate amounts of metabolic energy for the cells can break down due to a severe lack of oxygen or to poisoning. When this happens, the Na^+ pump fails and the cells take up Na^+ through passive diffusion. Consequently, as was described in the preceding section, the membrane potential declines, the ionic distributions inside and outside the cell balance each other, and the cells swell. They soon become incapable of functioning and finally suffer irreversible damage. Therefore an adequately functioning Na^+ pump is vitally important for the existence of the cells.

The coupled Na^+-K^+ pump. The extracellular K^+ concentration also has a strong influence on the active Na^+ transport. In the absence of extracellular K^+, the Na^+ efflux falls to about 30 percent of its normal value. The reason for this dependence of the Na^+ efflux on the K^+ concentration is to be found in an *exchange process*: For each Na^+ ion transported out of the cell, a K^+ ion can be taken into the cell. This exchange process is called a *coupled Na^+-K^+ pump*. The model in Fig. 2-8 was developed to show how the coupled pump operates. It can be seen that intracellular Na^+ ions bind themselves to a carrier molecule Y on the inner side of the membrane. The NaY complex can diffuse through the membrane. At the outer side of the membrane the complex breaks down spontaneously so that the external concentration of NaY becomes less than the inner concentration. Consequently, the efflux of the NaY exceeds the influx. Thus, by temporarily combining with the carrier molecule Y, the Na^+ diffuses against its concentration and potential gradients.

On the outside of the membrane, carrier molecule Y is converted by an enzyme into carrier molecule X. X combines with extracellular K^+ to form KX, and in this form diffuses to the inside. Here, KX, in turn, breaks down, having effected the transport of K^+ as well as the migration of X to the inside of the membrane. Finally, on the inside of the membrane, the carrier molecule X is converted back into carrier molecule Y with the expenditure of energy and is then available once more for the Na^+ transport cycle. In this reaction model the conversion of carrier molecule X into carrier molecule Y is the active step in the transport process.

The NaY complex is usually electrically neutral. As a result, during the transport process no electric charge is transferred through the membrane, and the membrane potential is unaffected by the transport process itself. This *sodium pump* is therefore also termed *electrically neutral*. The mechanism of the coupled Na^+-K^+ pump probably developed because it *saves metabolic energy*. For the operation of the Na^+ pump, cells require considerable amounts of metabolic energy. It

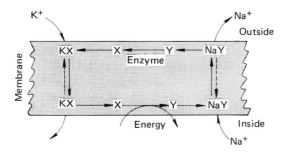

Fig. 2-8. Coupled Na^+-K^+ pump. Diagram of the transport of Na^+ and K^+ through the membrane with the aid of carrier molecules Y and X. See text for further details. (From Glynn: *Progr. Biophys.* **8**, 241, 1958.)

is estimated that *10 to 20 percent of the resting metabolism* of a muscle cell is *expended for the active transport of Na⁺*. This energy requirement would be higher were it not for the fact that the greater part of the Na^+ transport is accomplished by a coupled Na^+-K^+ pump. With a coupled pump, no energy is consumed during the return of the carrier molecule to the inside of the cells, and the energy actually consumed is about half that required for uncoupled Na^+ transport.

Summary of ionic currents through the membrane.   Figure 2-9 summarizes the most important ionic currents (with the exception of Cl^-) through the membrane. This diagram of the membrane shows channels for the various ion movements in each direction. The width of the ion channels corresponds to the *magnitude* of the ionic current flowing through them, and their slope corresponds to the *driving potential* for the ionic current in question. The potential between inside and outside, namely, the *resting potential*, is taken to be -80 mV.

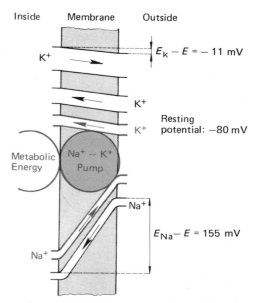

Fig. 2-9.   Passive and active ion movements through the membrane. In the diagram the width of the channels for the various ionic currents indicates the magnitude of the current, and the slope of the channels indicates the driving force behind the ionic current. The Na^+-K^+ pump enables the Na^+ and K^+ currents (colored red) to flow against the direction of the driving force. (From Eccles: *The Physiology of Nerve Cells*, Baltimore, Johns Hopkins Press, 1957.)

Consider first the movement of the K^+ *ions*. The resting potential here is 11 mV less negative than the K^+ equilibrium potential; therefore the K^+ ions are driven to the outside by this driving potential of 11 mV. This is why the K^+ channels are slightly sloping to the outside. The passive K^+ efflux (uppermost in diagram) therefore outweighs the passive K^+ influx, and more K^+ ions can diffuse "downhill" than "uphill." The difference between the passive K^+ currents is made up by active K^+ transport. Like all active processes in Fig. 2-9, the active K^+ transport into the cell is colored red, and the "active K^+ channel" is also connected to the pump driven by metabolic energy.

Active transport accounts for only a small portion of the K^+ currents. In contrast, practically all the *Na^+ efflux* from the cell is achieved by the *Na^+ pump*. The deviation of the resting potential from the sodium equilibrium potential, and thus the driving potential for the Na^+ ions, is very large (155 mV in Fig. 2-9). The "sodium channels" therefore are very steeply inclined toward the inside. The large driving potential greatly promotes passive sodium influx (bottom channel in Fig. 2-9) and practically blocks passive Na^+ efflux. (This is so negligible that it cannot be indicated in Fig. 2-9.) The passive Na^+ influx is in equilibrium with the active Na^+ efflux. In the "active Na^+ channel," the Na^+ ions are driven "uphill" by the pump. Overall, the Na^+ channels through the membrane are much narrower than the K^+ channels; therefore, despite large driving potentials, much less Na^+ than K^+ flows through the membrane. This reflects the low membrane conductance for Na^+ ions as compared to K^+.

Answer the following questions to check whether you have assimilated the information given thus far in the chapter.

Q 2.8   The Na^+ efflux from the cell is "active" because:
    a. The driving potential for the Na^+ efflux is large.
    b. No passive net Na^+ efflux can take place against the driving potential.
    c. Metabolic energy is required for the Na^+ efflux.
    d. The sodium conductance of the membrane is much higher than the potassium conductance.
    e. The sodium conductance of the membrane is much lower than the potassium conductance.

Q 2.9   Active Na^+ transport can be blocked or greatly reduced by
    a. Lowering the extracellular K^+ concentration.
    b. Lowering the intracellular K^+ concentration.
    c. Increasing the intracellular Na^+ concentration.
    d. Cooling the cell.
    e. Poisoning the cell with DNP.

Q 2.10 At constant resting potential the passive sodium inflow is equal
to the
a. Passive potassium inflow.
b. Passive net potassium flow.
c. Active sodium outflow.
d. Active potassium outflow.

2.4   The Action Potential

The resting potential is the precondition for nerve cells and muscle fibers to be able to fulfill their specific functions in the body. It is
the task of nerve cells to pick up information, to transmit it throughout
the body, and to coordinate and integrate it. Muscle cells contract in
accordance with instructions received from nerves. When the cells
work and are "active" like this, short positive changes in the membrane potential occur. These changes are called "*action potentials.*"
The generation and the time course of such action potentials are
described below.

Time course of action potentials.   *Action potentials* can be measured in nerves and muscle cells by *intracellular electrodes.* The same
apparatus and procedure shown in Fig. 2-1 can be used to measure the
resting potential. As will be shown later (see page 60), the action
potentials can also be recorded by extracellular electrodes placed near
the cell. However, this procedure usually permits only an approximate determination of the time course of the action potential.

Figure 2-10 shows action potentials measured with intracellular
electrodes in vertebrate nerves, muscle cells, and cardiac muscle
cells. In all these action potentials, the potential, starting from the
resting potential, jumps very rapidly to a positive value and then
returns more slowly to the resting potential. The *peak* of the action
potential for all the examples shown is located somewhere near +30
mV. On the other hand, the *duration* of the action potential is very
different in the various types of cell. In the case of the nerve the
action potential lasts approximately 1 msec only, while in the cardiac
muscle it lasts more than 200 msec.

The terms for the various *phases of the action potential* are given
in Fig. 2-11. The action potential begins with a very rapid positive
change in potential, called *the upstroke* or *rising phase.* In nerves and
muscle cells of warm-blooded animals the upstroke lasts only 0.2 to
0.5 msec. During the upstroke, the cell loses its negative resting
charge or polarization. Therefore the upstroke of the action potential
is also called the *"depolarization phase."*

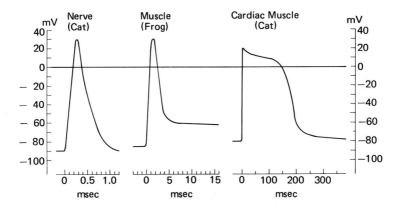

Fig. 2-10. Action potentials of various types of cells measured by intracellular electrodes. Abscissa: Time after start of action potential. Ordinate: Membrane potential. The time scale of the action potentials varies considerably. The nerve action potential of the cat is much shorter then the muscle action potential of the frog, and both are short relative to the action potential of the cardiac muscle.

In most types of cells the depolarization goes beyond zero to positive potentials. The positive portion of the action potential is referred to as the *overshoot*. Once the peak is reached, the action potential returns again to the resting potential. This process is called *"repolarization"* because the normal polarization of the cell membrane is restored.

Toward the end of the action potential the repolarization slows down in many types of cells, and at the end of repolarization the potential may exceed the resting value in a negative direction for a

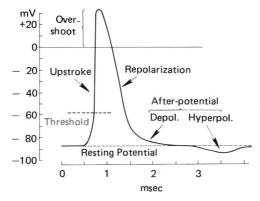

Fig. 2-11. Phases of the action potential. Diagram of the time course of a nerve action potential as shown in Fig. 2-10. The names of the various phases of the action potential are discussed in detail in the text.

certain time. These potential patterns at the end of or after repolarization are called *after-potentials* (see Fig. 2-11). If, at the end of the action potential, the membrane potential remains slightly more positive than the resting potential for a certain time, this is referred to as a *depolarizing after-potential.* If, on the other hand, the membrane potential goes beyond the value of the resting potential for a certain time, this is referred to as a *hyperpolarizing after-potential.* A well-developed after-potential is seen in Fig. 2-10 in the action potential of the frog muscle.

Triggering of the action potential and excitation. According to what has been said so far, the resting potential is a constant and stable state. What event must occur for this stable state to be disrupted, thus triggering an action potential? Action potentials are generated whenever the membrane, starting from the resting potential, is depolarized to approximately −50 mV. The processes that bring about this initial depolarization will be discussed later (see page 53). The potential from which the action potential starts is called the *threshold* (see Fig. 2-11). The *membrane charge is unstable* at this threshold potential. The charge dissipates rapidly and automatically and usually even reverses its polarity. This results in the rapid upstroke of the action potential that goes beyond the zero potential (the overshoot phase).

The condition of a spontaneous, progressive discharge of the membrane that is triggered at the threshold is also called *excitation.* The excitation lasts only a short while, usually less than 1 msec. It is thus comparable to an explosion that dies away very quickly.

The depolarization phase of the action potential itself sets processes in motion that restore the resting membrane charge. The excitation-induced depolarization phase of the action potential is followed by a spontaneous repolarization to the resting potential. The stereotyped, cyclic sequence of the action potential can be compared with the operating cycle of a cylinder in an internal combustion engine: an ignition spark heats the gas mixture to a level (corresponding to the threshold of the action potential) at which it explodes (corresponding to excitation). In turn, the explosion sets off mechanisms that restore the system to the state that existed before the explosion (corresponding to repolarization); exhaust gases are expelled, and fresh gas mixture is drawn in and compressed.

Definition of the action potential. The action potential in each cell is a stereotyped sequence of depolarization and repolarization of the membrane that occurs spontaneously whenever the membrane is depolarized beyond the threshold potential. Cells in which action

potentials can be triggered are called *"excitable."* Excitability is a
typical property of nerve and muscle cells.

Action potentials in a particular cell always follow a constant sequence. It makes little difference how the threshold is reached by the
initial depolarization, nor does it matter whether the initial depolarizing process itself exceeds the threshold to a greater or lesser extent.
This constant nature of the action potential is also called the
"all-or-nothing" law of excitation.

Ion shifts occurring during the action potential.   If the membrane
potential undergoes a strong change even to positive values during
the action potential, then the charge of the membrane capacitor also
has to change and ions have to be displaced across the membrane. The
type and extent of these ionic shifts will be discussed with the aid of
Fig. 2-12. The parts printed in black are a repeat of Fig. 2-2, which
showed the ion distribution over a small area of the cell membrane
and its surroundings at the resting potential. The *resting potential*
was characterized by a *high* K^+ *conductance* of the membrane. Be-

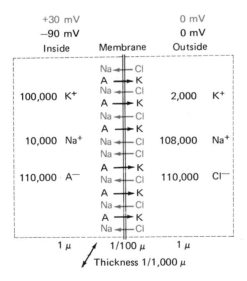

Fig. 2-12.   Reversal of membrane charge during excitation. Same diagram
as Fig. 2-2 but showing the charge conditions during excitation. The membrane charge is given for the small area of $1 \mu \times 1/1000 \mu$ and the number of
ions is given for the two spaces, each $1 \mu \times 1 \mu \times 1/1000 \mu$ volume, on either
side of the membrane. The pairs of ions attached to the membrane during the
resting potential are shown in black and the change in membrane charge
during excitation is shown in red. During excitation an excess of 2 Na^+ occurs
inside the membrane; this corresponds to a membrane potential of +30 mV.

cause of the concentration gradient, K^+ ions flowed out of the cell until the resulting membrane charge prevented any further efflux. This state of equilibrium was reached in the example in Figs. 2-2 and 2-12 when the membrane became charged with 6 K^+ and the corresponding number of A^-, giving rise to a "resting potential" of −90 mV.

It is a property of the membrane that when it is depolarized to the region of the threshold potential, its *conductance for Na$^+$ ions, g_{Na}, increases.* As a result, Na^+ ions (printed in red in Fig. 2-12) flow into the cell. The Na^+ ions that flow into the cell partly compensate for the resting charge, that is, the potential becomes less negative. As a result of this depolarization, g_{Na} increases still further, and more Na^+ ions flow into the cell. g_{Na} finally attains more than 100 times its resting value; that is to say, *during excitation g_{Na} becomes greater than g_K.* If the condition of increased g_{Na} is maintained long enough, the membrane charge is reversed. During excitation, however, the membrane potential can attain no more than the Na^+ equilibrium potential, for at this potential the positive membrane potential balances the inward-directed osmotic pressure arising from the concentration difference for Na^+ ions. The Na^+ equilibrium potential is situated at approximately +60 mV. At this potential an excess of 4 Na^+ should exist at the inner side of the membrane in the example in Fig. 2-12. Therefore, in order to compensate for the six anions located on the inner side of the membrane at the resting potential, a total of 10 Na^+ should flow into the cell until the Na^+ equilibrium potential is reached.

In accordance with the description just given of the Na^+ inward current during excitation, the peak of the action potential should be situated at the Na^+ equilibrium potential, at approximately +60 mV. As Fig. 2-10 has shown, the peaks of the action potentials are situated at +30 mV and thus do not reach the Na^+ equilibrium potential. There are two reasons for this: first, the *increase in Na$^+$ conductance does not last long enough* to permit the reversal of the membrane charge to go quite as far as E_{Na}. In the diagram given in Fig. 2-12, not 10 but only 8 Na^+ ions have time to flow inward; this creates an excess of only 2 Na^+ ions at the inner side of the membrane, which, in turn, generates a peak potential of +30 mV.

The second reason why E_{Na} is not attained by the peak of the action potential is that the depolarization of the membrane, along with the described increase in g_{Na}, also *gives a powerful boost to the K$^+$ conductance g_K of the membrane, but with a lag of not quite 1 msec.* Thus, when the peak of the action potential is reached less than 1 msec after the start of excitation, the *K$^+$ ions* begin to flow *out of the cell* in increased numbers and rapidly compensate for the influx of positive charges in the form of Na^+ ions. Finally, g_K becomes larger than g_{Na}, the efflux of positive charges outweighs the influx, and the membrane charge becomes more negative. This predominant K^+ *efflux* causes the *repolarization phase* of the action potential. In the nerves of warm-blooded animals, the inner side of the membrane once more acquires a full negative charge, and the resting potential is restored about 1 msec after the start of excitation.

The *ionic movements* during the action potential may be *summarized* as follows: as a result of depolarization beyond the threshold, the Na^+ conductance increases rapidly; the K^+ conductance also increases but with a time lag. Therefore, initially Na^+ ions flow rapidly into the cell, and the membrane potential moves in the direction of the Na^+ equilibrium potential at +60mV; then K^+ ions flow out of the cell, restoring the resting membrane charge and repolarizing the membrane to the resting potential.

Ionic shifts during the action potential. Despite the large changes in the conductance of the membrane during the action potential the ionic shifts through the membrane are *small* in relation to the quantities of ions surrounding the membrane. In the diagram in Fig. 2-12 only 8 Na^+ ions need to flow in during excitation; similarly, repolarization would be achieved by the efflux of 6 K^+ ions. As a result of these ion shifts, the Na^+ concentration in the very small spaces adjoining the cell (see Fig. 2-12) would vary by less than 1/1,000 during an action potential.

The Na^+ ions that flowed into the cell with the action potential are expelled again in the course of time by the Na^+ pump. The active Na^+ transport compensates for not only the resting sodium influx but also the Na^+ influx during excitation. However, the active Na^+ transport is of no importance for the individual action potentials. If the ion pump is blocked, for example, by poisoning with dinitrophenol (see page 30), then, despite the fact that active transport has been eliminated, thousands of action potentials can occur before the intracellular Na^+ concentration becomes so high that the cell is rendered inexcitable. The action potential thus arises from *passive* movements of the ions along their concentration gradients. Energy-consuming processes such as the Na^+ pump are only necessary insofar as they maintain the concentration gradients.

The action potential and Na^+ deficiency. The role of the Na^+ ions in the excitation process can be demonstrated by a simple experiment. If the extracellular Na^+ concentration is slowly reduced (while balancing out the osmolarity), the resting potential, as discussed above, remains practically unchanged. Usually it becomes about 10 mV more negative (see page 26). On the other hand, the action potential is clearly affected: the peak potential, that is, the action potential over-shoot, becomes less positive, and the upstroke becomes slower. If the extracellular Na^+ concentration drops to about one-tenth of the nor-mal, that is, below 20 mM, the cells finally become *inexcitable*. The reason for this is that during excitation under normal conditions a strong Na^+ influx depolarizes the cell, and this influx is now reduced because the extracellular Na^+ concentration is too low. The high intracellular K^+ concentration is a precondition for the *resting poten-tial* while a high extracellular Na^+ concentration is necessary for the *action potential*. In addition, excitability is also dependent on a low intracellular Na^+ concentration so that Na^+ can flow into the cell.

Answer the following questions to check whether you have fully mastered the material dealt with in this section.

Q 2.11 Draw the action potential of a nerve with amplitude and time scales. Name the various phases.

Q 2.12 Which of the following statements apply to the threshold of the action potential?
   a. The membrane potential is positive and close to E_{Na}.
   b. The membrane potential is approximately 20–30 mV more positive than the resting potential.
   c. The membrane charge is unstable and dissipates spontane-ously.
   d. The potassium efflux is larger than the sodium influx.

Q 2.13 The repolarization of the action potential is brought about by the
   a. very small increase in the intracellular Na^+ concentration caused by excitation.
   b. potassium efflux, which sets in with a time lag after de-polarization.
   c. termination of the sodium influx during excitation.
   d. expulsion of the Na^+ influx by the sodium pump.

2.5   Kinetics of Excitation

The action potential is caused by a Na^+ current flowing into the cell and a K^+ current then flowing out, both events being caused by depolarization beyond the threshold. These currents depend on the extent of the depolarization as well as on the time that elapses from the initiation of depolarization. The complicated kinetics of these Na^+ and K^+ currents will now be discussed in detail. This knowledge is not only useful for further analysis of the action potential but is in fact necessary for a full understanding of how the action potential is propagated and the events through which the threshold of the action potential is reached.

Measuring the potential dependence and time dependence of the ionic currents.   The sodium and potassium currents that flow during the action potential are strongly dependent on potential and time. Because the potential changes rapidly throughout the action potential, the potential dependence of the currents cannot be analyzed in more detail during the action potential itself. Such an analysis can be performed, however, if the potential of the cell is held constant artificially after the onset of excitation. An experimental set up that enables this is called a *voltage clamp*.

Figure 2-13 illustrates such a voltage clamp. In this experiment two intracellular electrodes are used. With one electrode the *membrane potential is measured* in the manner already described in Fig. 2-1. The second intracellular electrode supplies current to the cell. The two electrodes are connected to an electronic regulating device. The apparatus can be programmed in such a way that the membrane potential changes suddenly from one value to another and remains constant there. The regulating device ensures that exactly the right amount of current flows through the current electrode to induce the change in potential, and that once the potential has been changed the current through the electrode is adjusted so that the new membrane potential remains constant. If, for example, the change in potential

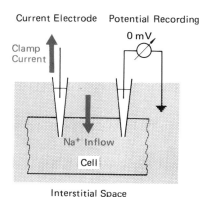

Fig. 2-13.   Voltage clamp currents. The membrane potential between the inside of the cell and the interstitial space is measured by the electrode on the right. The clamp current (red arrow pointing upward), which maintains the potential at 0 mV, flows out of the cell through the left electrode. The clamp current is of the same magnitude, but of opposite polarity, as the Na^+ inflow (red arrow pointing downward) through the cell membrane at the clamp potential 0 mV.

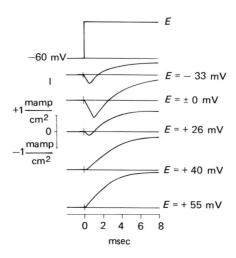

Fig. 2-14. Clamp currents following changes in potential. The top line shows the time course of a potential change in a giant axon of a squid starting from a resting potential of −60 mV to clamp potential E. Below that are the clamp currents that flow after the potential change to the potential E, as shown to the right of the curves in each case. The calibration of the clamp current as given for the potential jump to +26 mV is also valid for the other clamp currents. Positive clamp currents correspond to an outflow of positive ions from the cell, and negative clamp currents correspond to an inflow of positive ions. (From Hodgkin and Huxley: *J. Physiol.* **116**, 449, 1952.)

involves a suprathreshold depolarization starting from the resting potential, this will trigger a Na^+ inflow. In this case the regulator will allow just enough current to leave the cell to balance the inflow of Na^+ ions (see Fig. 2-13). As both currents cancel out each other, the membrane potential remains constant. The clamp current and its time course are measured. Since it is always just big enough to cancel out the membrane current, it is an exact mirror image of the membrane currents. Thus, at a constant *clamp potential* the *clamp current* indicates the *time course of the ionic currents* through the membrane at this potential.

Membrane currents after a depolarization.   In 1952 Hodgkin and Huxley published a pioneering analysis of the action potential of the *giant axon of squid* using the voltage-clamp technique.* Because of the large fiber diameter of up to 1 mm, this particular preparation is especially suitable for such studies, and since 1952 it has been the subject of continuing research. Figure 2-14 illustrates the clamp cur-

*J. Physiol. **116**, 449 (1952).

rents measured in such a fiber. The top trace of the figure represents the programmed jump in potential from the resting potential at -60 mV to the value E. The traces below this indicate the clamp currents measured at the various values for potential E.

In the case of the smallest jump to $E = -33$ mV, a small negative current flows for about 1 msec following depolarization. This negative current then changes into a steady positive current. If the cell is depolarized to 0 mV, then both the short-duration negative and the subsequent steadily positive current components become larger. When the cell is further depolarized to $+26$ mV, the initial negative current component then becomes smaller, and it disappears entirely at $E = +40$ mV. When still further depolarization occurs to $+55$ mV, a positive current component takes the place of the hitherto negative one. While the initial current becomes smaller at potentials above 0 mV and finally reverses its direction, the later positive current continues to increase with depolarization.

The reversal of polarity at $+40$ mV identifies this *initial current as a sodium current*, for in the case of the giant axons of squid, E_{Na} is situated at $+40$ mV. *Beyond its equilibrium potential an ionic current must reverse its direction.* At potentials more negative than E_{Na}, sodium ions flow into the cell; at potentials more positive than E_{Na}, sodium ions flow out of the cell. The initial negative clamp current can also be identified by further measurement as Na^+ current. If Na^+ is replaced in the extracellular solution by a nonpermeable ion (see page 28), this current component disappears completely because there is no Na^+ current in the sodium-free solution. In suprathreshold depolarizations to a fixed potential, a *sodium current* flows for 1 to 2 msec.

The positive current following the Na^+ current after a depolarization step is a K^+ current. The time course of the K^+ current is clearly visible at $E = +40$ mV, the Na^+ equilibrium potential E_{Na}. At E_{Na} there is, by definition, no net Na^+ flow; therefore current measured at that potential must be all K^+ current. In contrast to the sodium current, I_{Na}, which sets in immediately but flows for only a short time, the potassium current I_K starts with a *delay*, attains its maximum in 4 to 10 msec, and *does not decline* provided the depolarization is maintained. The amplitude of maximum I_K increases approximately in proportion to the depolarization.

As discussed above, the sodium inflow after depolarization does not take place in a sodium-free solution. The membrane currents which are then measured after a depolarization step are (essentially) K^+ currents. Thus the time course of the current can be determined for each potential. If this K^+ current is subtracted from the current measured in a normal bath solution, we get the sodium current. So it is possible to separate the clamp current at each membrane potential into the Na⁺ and the K⁺ components. This has been done in Fig. 2-15 for E = 0 mV. The figure shows clearly how I_{Na} rises almost without delay after depolarization and drops again after less than 1 msec. I_K, on the other hand, increases with a time lag to a constant end value.

Changes in membrane conductance following depolarization. The changes in *membrane conductance* give a better indication than the membrane currents of the behavior of the membrane following depolarization and during the action potential. At a given potential E the membrane conductance for an ion is proportional to the ionic current through the membrane. In the case of Na⁺, for example, we can write:

$$g_{Na} = I_{Na}/(E - E_{Na})$$

If the equilibrium potentials E_{Na} and E_K are known, then for a given potential E, one can calculate the time course of g_{Na} and g_K from the time course of I_{Na} and I_K. The former time course is shown for $E = 0$ mV in the bottom trace in Fig. 2-15. g_{Na} reaches its maximum in less than 1 msec after depolarization and has almost disappeared after about 4 msec, although the depolarized state continues. This latter condition is called *inactivation*.

The inactivation of the g_{Na}, which rose following depolarization,

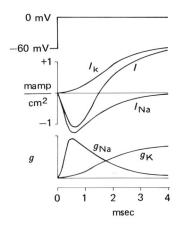

Fig. 2-15. Ion currents and conductance following a change in potential. Top: Time course of the change in potential induced by the voltage clamp from −60 to 0 mV. Center: Clamp current I and its components I_{Na} and I_K flowing after the change in potential. Bottom: The time courses for membrane conductances g_{Na} and g_K calculated from these currents. Preparation: giant axon of squid. (From Hodgkin: *Proc. Roy. Soc.* **B148**, 1, 1958.)

continues for as long as the membrane remains depolarized. Once g_{Na} has been *inactivated* after a depolarization, it is *not available for activation by further depolarization.* The sodium system can recover from inactivation only when the membrane potential returns to the vicinity of the resting potential or to still more negative potentials. In order to permit the inactivated sodium system to become *available for activation* again, the membrane potential must remain more negative than −50 mV for one to several milliseconds. Consequently, the sodium system is available for activation by a depolarization only if the membrane potential has had a sufficiently negative value for at least several milliseconds prior to depolarization. At resting potentials more positive than −50 mV, g_{Na} remains inactivated in the nerves of warm-blooded animals, and therefore no excitation can be triggered from this potential range.

The sodium system can exist in any of three different potential-dependent and time-dependent states: (1) available for activation at potentials more negative than −50 mV; (2) activated following supra-threshold depolarizations, but only for a few msec; (3) inactivated after several milliseconds at potentials more positive than −50 mV. The transition from activation to inactivation is dependent on time, and the transition from inactivation to availability for activation is dependent on repolarization and time.

In contrast to g_{Na}, g_K *does not become inactivated during depolarization.* As Fig. 2-15 shows, g_K remains increased following a depolarization for as long as the depolarization lasts. Since the rise in g_K is responsible for the repolarization of the resting potential, the high g_K, which does not decline during depolarization, definitely guarantees the return of the potential to the resting value.

Membrane conductance during the action potential. If the dependence of the membrane conductance on potential and time is known for certain fixed clamp potentials, then it is also possible to calculate the time course of g_{Na} and g_K during the action potential. The result of such a calculation is shown in Fig. 2-16. g_{Na} increases sharply as a function of potential at the start of the action potential and reaches its *maximum before the peak of the action potential* (dotted vertical line in Fig. 2-16). After attaining its maximum, g_{Na} declines, at first because of the time-dependent inactivation and, when the membrane is nearly repolarized, also because of its potential dependence. At the beginning of the action potential, triggered by depolarization, g_K can *rise only slowly* because of its time dependence, and it reaches its maximum during the steepest section of the repolarization phase. After this it declines slowly because of its *potential dependence.*

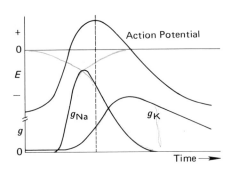

Fig. 2-16. Membrane conductance during action potential. Top: Time course of an action potential. Below: The time courses of membrane conductances g_{Na} and g_K during the action potential. (From Noble: *Physiol. Rev.* **46**, 1, 1966.)

Refractory phases following the action potential. Already at the peak of the action potential g_{Na} is partly inactivated, and this inactivation is more or less complete by the time the repolarization intersects the zero line. The inactivation can be reversed and the sodium system can once again become available for activation only when the potential remains more negative than -50 mV for several msec (see page 45). g_{Na} is thus inactivated during repolarization of the action potential as well as for a short time afterward. During this time g_{Na} cannot be substantially increased by a new depolarization; that is, the cell is *inexcitable.*

The phase of inexcitability following the action potential can also be detected by depolarizing the membrane potential to the threshold at various times following the action potential, in this way determining the excitability. The result of such an experiment is shown in Fig. 2-17. The induced depolarization of the cell is indicated by the broken curves. The cell is seen to be absolutely *inexcitable* in the first 2 msec following the start of the action potential. No matter how large the depolarizations, the threshold cannot be reached. This phase of complete inexcitability is also called the *absolute refractory period.*

Figure 2-17 also shows that for a few milliseconds after the end of the absolute refractory period the threshold for the triggering of action potentials is located at values more positive than for the first action potential. The period up to the time when the threshold returns to normal is called the *relative refractory period.* The amplitude of the action potential is also reduced during this phase because the sodium system has not fully recovered from the inactivation following the first action potential.

The absolute refractory period limits the maximum frequency at which action potentials can be triggered in the cell. If, as in Fig. 2-17,

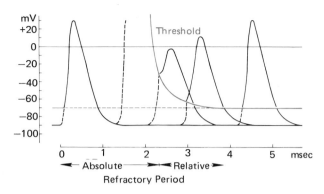

Fig. 2-17. Refractoriness following excitation. Diagram of the time course of an action potential in the nerve of a warm-blooded animal following triggering of further action potentials at different times. The solid red line denotes the threshold. The broken black curves denote in each case the depolarization of the fiber to the threshold. The solid black curves represent the spontaneous courses of the potentials once the threshold is exceeded. The fiber is inexcitable during the absolute refractory period after the first action potential. No matter how large the depolarization, the threshold cannot be reached. The threshold is higher than normal (thin broken line) in the subsequent relative refractory period.

the absolute refractory period ends 2 msec after the start of the action potential, then the *maximum frequency of the action potentials* in this cell is 500/sec. There are cells with even shorter refractory periods, so that in an extreme case frequencies up to 1,000/sec can occur in a nerve. In most types of cells, however, the maximum action potential frequencies measured are below 500/sec.

The following questions will help you check the knowledge you have acquired.

Q 2.14 At the peak of the action potential the membrane potential becomes positive because:
  a. The Na^+ concentration in the cell becomes larger than the K^+ concentration.
  -b. A Na^+ influx generates a slight excess of positive charges on the inside of the membrane.
  c. The membrane potential becomes more positive than the Na^+ equilibrium potential.
  d. The membrane potential approaches the Na^+ equilibrium potential.

Q 2.15 During the steep phase of repolarization, what flows through the membrane?
  a. Mainly Na^+ current.
  b. Mainly K^+ current.
  c. Na^+ and K^+ currents of approximately the same magnitude.

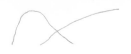

Q 2.16 Plot the approximate time course of g_{Na} and g_K during the action
potential.

Q 2.17 During the absolute refractory phase after an action potential
the
  → a. cell is inexcitable.
    b. sodium inflow is greater than the potassium outflow.
  → e. sodium conductance is not available for activation.
    d. sodium pump is not active.
    e. sodium equilibrium potential is negative.

2.6   Electrotonus and Stimulus

Excitation occurs as a result of depolarization of the membrane to
the threshold. The actual process of excitation was discussed in detail
in the preceding sections, but nothing has been said so far about how
the membrane is depolarized to the threshold. This depolarization is
also called *stimulation*, and this section will deal with the characteristics of such stimuli.

In the cells that make up the body the *stimulus* that triggers an
action potential is usually an electric current that depolarizes the cell.
Normally, this current is not generated in the region of the membrane
to be stimulated but comes from somewhere beyond that region. In
the case of nerve cells the stimulating current comes from neighboring sections of the nerve membrane, from synapses, or from receptors.
In neurophsiological experiments the stimulating current is usually
supplied by electrodes because this makes it easy to control its magnitude and duration. In this section, therefore, we will first discuss the
reaction of the membrane to an applied current and then analyze the
conditions under which such a current acts as a stimulus.

Electrotonus in the case of homogeneous current distribution. Fig.
2-18A shows how current can be fed into a cell through an intracellular electrode. The applied current, I, leaves the cell again by crossing
the membrane. It flows first via the *membrane capacity* and second as
ionic current through the membrane. In the process the membrane
potential, E, is changed. During and shortly after the end of the
current flow, the measuring electrode records an *electrotonic
potential*.

Let us first consider the current component that flows via the
membrane capacity. Depending on their polarity, the excess charges
that are introduced into the cell with the applied current can increase
or reduce the negative charge on the inner side of the membrane. An
inflow of positive charges will reduce the negative charge on the inner

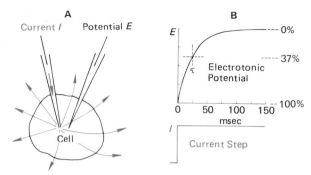

Fig. 2-18. Electrotonic potential of a spherical cell. *A*: Diagram showing measurement of potential *E* and of current supply *I* through intracellular electrodes. The current flow through the membrane is indicated by the red lines. *B*, Bottom: Time course of a current pulse *I* through the current electrode. Top: Time course of the simultaneously measured membrane potential *E*, the electrotonic potential. The gradient of the rise in the electrotonic potential is characterized by the membrane time constant τ, which is read off when the potential has approached to within 37 percent ($1/e$) of its final value.

side of the membrane (see Fig. 2-2). If the negative charge on the inner side of the membrane is reduced, then the positive charge on the outer side of the membrane declines correspondingly. Thus the number of positive charges released on the outer side of the membrane is equal to the number used up on the inside to reduce the negative charge, and there has been a current flow through the membrane although no carriers of charge have actually crossed the membrane. Since this current is generated by displacements of charge via the membrane capacity, it is called a *capacitative current, I_c*.

The membrane potential is proportional to the charge of the membrane capacitor. Given a constant supply of charge, that is, when a constant current is applied, the charge of the membrane capacitor, and as a result the *membrane potential*, should *change at a constant rate*. Figure 2-18*B* illustrates the changes in potential that occur in the cell following application of a constant current. The potential does not, in fact, change at a constant rate; instead, the rate of change decreases with time, and the potential finally attains a constant value despite the fact that current continues to flow. The time course of the change in potential must therefore be determined by more than just the flow of a *capacitative* current.

During the change in potential an *ionic current* flows in addition to the capacitative current. At the resting potential the membrane is particularly permeable to K^+ ions, less so to Cl^- ions, and only slightly to Na^+ ions. At constant resting potential, the sum of these ionic currents is zero. If the membrane potential is shifted by charges supplied through an electrode, a net ionic current flows that is proportional to the magnitude of the shift in potential. This is because the ionic currents are proportional to the membrane conductance and vary in proportion to the difference between the membrane potential and the equilibrium potential. If, as in Fig. 2-18B, the membrane charge is reduced by a constant current, then with increasing displacement from the resting potential more ionic current will flow across the membrane. This current is mainly carried by K$^+$ ions. As depolarization increases, less and less current is available for discharging the membrane capacitor. Consequently, the membrane potential changes more and more slowly with time until it finally becomes constant when all the applied current flows through the membrane as ionic current I_i.

The exponential time course of the electrotonic potential as shown in Fig. 2-18 is the result. At the start of this electrotonic potential, nothing but capacitative current flows through the membrane, but at the plateau the current is entirely ionic current. This state is characterized not only by the magnitude of the plateau, that is, the amplitude of the electrotonic potential, but also by the steepness of the exponential increase. This, in turn, is characterized by the *membrane time constant* τ, that is, the time required for the potential to reach 37 percent ($1/e$) of its final amplitude. The value for τ varies for different membranes, ranging from 10 to 50 msec.

Measurements of electrotonic potentials are used often in neurophysiology to determine the resistance and capacity of the membrane. The *membrane resistance, r_m,* of a cell is the quotient of the final amplitude of the electrotonic potential and the applied current. At the plateau of the electrotonic potential the entire current flows as ionic current across the membrane resistance, and the latter can be calculated from the change in potential and the current. The time course of the electrotonic potential represents the curve for the charging of the membrane capacitor across the membrane resistance, and the membrane time constant, τ, is the product of resistance and capacitance. The *membrane capacity, c_m,* can thus be calculated as the quotient of τ and r_m. These simple relationships only hold true, however, for cells in which the applied current is distributed homogeneously.

Electrotonic potential in elongated cells.   Almost all nerve fibers and muscle cells are very long in relation to their diameter. A nerve fiber, for example, can be 1 meter long with a diameter of 1 μ. In these cells, current applied at one point naturally flows through the membrane at much greater density in the vicinity of this point than in more distant parts of the membrane. Therefore the electrotonic potentials in such cells must be governed by quite different conditions from those in spherical cells (Fig. 2-18A) where the current is distributed homogeneously.

As shown in Fig. 2-19, the *electrotonic potentials* in an elongated muscle fiber can be measured by inserting intracellular electrodes at various distances—here at 0 mm, 2.5 mm, and 5 mm—from the current electrode. The *time course* measured for the *electrotonic potential* is *no longer simply exponential*, as in the case of the spherical cell shown in Fig. 2-18. At the site of current application the electrotonic potential (E_0) in Fig. 2-19 rises more steeply than when the current is evenly distributed. This is evident from the fact that at the moment when the membrane time constant, τ, is reached the electrotonic potential is already within 16 percent instead of 37 percent of its final value.

This more rapid increase is due to the inhomogeneous distribution

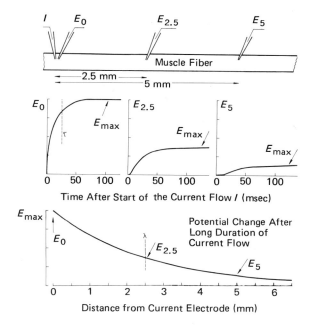

Fig. 2-19. Electrotonic potential in an elongated cell. Top: Diagram showing the application of current I in an elongated muscle fiber and the measuring of the change in potential, the electrotonic potential, at 0 mm (E_0), 2.5 mm ($E_{2.5}$), and 5 mm (E_5) from the site of current application. Center: Time courses of electrotonic potentials E_0, $E_{2.5}$, and E_5. With increasing distance the electrotonic potentials attain smaller final values E_{max}. Bottom: Final values, E_{max}, plotted as a function of the distance from the point of current application. The gradient of the decline of E_{max} with distance is characterized by the membrane length constant, λ, which is read at the site where the electrotonic potential reaches 37 percent of E_0.

of the current: first the membrane capacitor is discharged in a small region close to the current electrode, and only then does current flow through the interior of the cell, which has a considerable longitudinal resistance, to more distant parts of the membrane. Thus, when the current pulse is first applied, the membrane current concentrates in the direct vicinity of the current electrode, and the potential undergoes a rapid change here. Therefore, the time course of the electrontonic potential becomes slower with increasing distance from the site of current application. As Fig. 2-19 shows, at a distance of 5 mm the electrotonic potential (E_5) starts with a delay, and after 120 msec it has still not quite attained its final value E_{max}.

Even when the applied current has been flowing for a long time and a new charge distribution is attained, more current still flows through the parts of the membrane close to the point where current is fed in than through more distant parts. The amplitudes E_{max} of the final values of the electrotonic potentials are plotted in Fig. 2-19 (bottom) against the distance from the current electrode. It can be seen that the amplitude of E_{max} falls exponentially with distance. The gradient of the exponential decline of E_{max} with distance is characterized by the *membrane length constant*, λ, at which E_{max} has declined to 37 percent ($1/e$). λ is 2.5 mm in Fig. 2-19. The value of λ varies in different cells from 0.1 to 5 mm. In the length constant λ we therefore have a yardstick for judging over what distances electrotonic potentials can spread in elongated cells. At the distance 4λ, for example, the amplitude of the electrotonic potential is only 1 percent of the value of the potential close to the point of current application. Thus, in nerves electrotonic potentials can really only be measured over distances up to a few centimeters away from their point of origin.

Electrotonic potentials as passive membrane reactions.   The electrotonic potential is a purely passive reaction of the membrane to applied current, that is, the membrane does *not* change its *conductance* (or its capacity) during the electrotonic potential. The polarity of the current is also, in principle, of no significance for the course of the electrotonic potential. Depending on whether positive or negative current is applied, depolarizing or hyperpolarizing electrotonic potentials are generated—the time course of the one being the mirror image of the other.

A depolarizing electrotonic potential is also called catelectrotonus and a hyperpolarizing electrotonic potential is called anelectrotonus. These terms are derived from the procedure of applying current through two extracellular electrodes in contact with the nerve: catelectrotonus is generated around the cathode and anelectrotonus around the anode.

However, undistorted electrotonic potentials can only be measured if they displace the membrane potential just to such an extent that it does not change the membrance conductance. If, for example, the excitation threshold is reached during a depolarizing electrotonic potential, the time course of the potential deviates greatly from that of a subthreshold electrotonic potential.

Suprathreshold electrotonic potentials and the strength-duration curve. When a depolarizing electrotonic potential crosses the threshold an excitation is triggered. The current pulse that generates such a change in potential is called a stimulating current, or *stimulus*. If the current is just sufficient to drive the electrotonic potential to the threshold, it is known as the minimum stimulating current. All currents that are stronger than this minimum stimulating current act as stimuli, and because of the all-or-nothing character of excitation they trigger action potentials of equal amplitude.

Both the *amplitude* of the stimulating current and the *duration for which it flows* are important in the generation of excitation. A stimulating current that is just sufficient to depolarize the membrane to the threshold generates an electrotonic potential that reaches the threshold only at its maximum value. In the case of the muscle cell in Fig. 2-19 (see time course at E_0) it does this after more than 50 msec. Given a stronger stimulating current, the generated electrotonic potential reaches the threshold earlier. The stimulating current therefore needs to flow for a shorter time. The relationship between stimulating current strength and minimum stimulus duration is shown in Fig. 2-20A for the same muscle cell as in Fig. 2-19. This relationship is called the *strength-duration curve*.

In the case of very strong stimuli the strength-duration curve approaches asymptotically the time zero, and in the case of longlasting stimuli it approaches asymptotically a minimum stimulating current. The stimulating current that is just large enough to trigger an excitation in the case of stimuli of extended duration is called the *rheobase I_R*. When the stimulus duration is shortened, the necessary current strength increases rapidly. The extent to which the stimulus current strength increases when the stimulus duration becomes shorter is characterized by the *chronaxie*. The chronaxie is the necessary *duration* of a stimulating current of twice rheobasic strength.

The *strength-duration curve* can be constructed from the course of the electrotonic potential at various stimulating currents, as has been done in Fig. 2-20B. For a given stimulating current strength, the duration of the stimulus is the time at which the electrotonic potential generated by the current reaches the threshold. The figure depicts electrotonic potentials (black) which were triggered by constant cur-

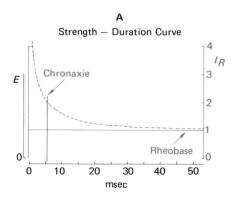

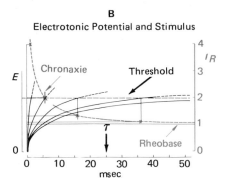

Fig. 2-20. Electrotonic potential and strength-duration curve. A: Strength-duration curve. The broken red curve shows the dependence of the threshold potential (or of the threshold current, right ordinate) on the stimulus duration (abscissa). The chronaxie is read at twice the rheobasic strength. B: Electrotonic potential and stimulus. Construction of the strength-duration curve (broken red curve) from the electrotonic potentials (black curves) that reach the threshold (broken black horizontal line) at different times, the stimulus durations, for various currents I (solid red lines). The currents I are given as multiples of the rheobase current strength I_R (right ordinate). See text for more details.

rent (red) of 1.1, 1.4, 2.0, and 4.0 times the rheobasic current strength, I_R. These electrotonic potentials reach the threshold at 36, 17, 6, and 1.5 msec, respectively. These stimulus durations are shown in the figure as crosses at the ordinate values of the appropriate currents. The curve joining these crosses is the strength-duration curve.

The *chronaxie* is a measure of the excitability of a cell. As can be seen from Fig. 2-20B, it is essentially determined by the steepness at which the electrotonic potentials rise; it is therefore proportional to the membrane time constant τ, which is the product of membrane resistance r_m and membrane capacity c_m (see page 50). If one of these values should vary, the chronaxie is affected proportionally. Furthermore, the chronaxie increases as the threshold potential becomes more positive.

Neurological applications of chronaxie measurements. As a measure of excitability the chronaxie has the advantage that it can be determined without knowing the absolute amplitude of the stimulating current for the cell. It is sufficient to measure the rheobase, the minimum current strength after a stimulus of extended duration. To measure the chronaxie, all that is necessary is to double the rheobasic current strength. Consequently the chronaxie can even be measured in situations where only a small, unknown but constant portion of the stimulating current flows into the cell to be stimulated. This can be done, for example, by placing electrodes on the surface of the arm over a nerve which is to be stimulated and by passing current through them. An effective stimulus, that is, one that reaches the threshold, is indicated by a twitching of the muscle served by the nerve in question. Then, by applying long-duration stimuli, the rheobasic current strength is first established, and the chronaxie is then determined as the minimum stimulus duration at twice rheobasic current strength.

The *chronaxie* is also suitable as a measure of excitability particularly in *clinical-diagnostic tests* in which the stimulating current cannot be applied by intracellular electrodes. In neurology the chronaxie is measured primarily to diagnose and to check the progress of various types of muscular paralysis. Normally, when current is applied to the skin, rheobases of 2 to 20 mamp are found. In almost all muscles of warm-blooded animals the chronaxie is less than 1 msec. In the case of disease or disruption of the motor nerves the chronaxie can rise sharply. In severe paralysis, values of 20 to 100 msec are recorded.

Check what you have learned by answering the following questions:

Q 2.18 Without looking at Figs. 2-18 to 20, draw the time course of the electrotonic potential of a spherical cell following application of a constant current to the cell.

Q 2.19 The final amplitude of the electrotonic potential (given homogeneous distribution of the current) is proportional to the
a. membrane capacity.
b. membrane resistance.
c. reciprocal of the membrane conductance.
d. applied current.
e. duration of current flow.

Q 2.20 In an elongated cell, how does the final amplitude of the electrotonic potential change with the distance from the site of current application?
a. It remains constant.
b. It increases in proportion to the distance.

  c. It decreases in proportion to the distance.
  d. It increases in proportion to the square of the distance.
  e. It decreases exponentially with the distance.

Q 2.21 A current pulse acts as a stimulus when
  a. the sum of stimulating current and sodium inflow is larger
     than the potassium outflow under resting conditions.
  b. it reduces the membrane capacity.
  c. it depolarizes the membrane potential beyond the threshold
     after 1 msec.
  d. it depolarizes the membrane potential beyond the thres-
     hold.
  e. it reversibly increases the potassium outflow.

2.7   Propagation of the Action Potential

We now come to a discussion of the actual task of the nerve fibers
and the membrane of the muscle fibers: the propagation of excitation.
Before this could be understood it was first necessary, in the preceding sections, to deal with the mechanism of excitation at the membrane. Then it was shown how changes in potential spread over the
length of a fiber as a result of currents flowing through the inside of
the fiber. To understand how the action potential is propagated, we
must now combine the knowledge we have acquired about excitation
and electrotonus.

Velocity of conduction of the action potential.   Let us proceed
from the simple observation that a nerve propagates action potentials.
If the action potential of a nerve fiber is measured at two points not too
close together, and if the nerve is stimulated at one end, then an action
potential appears first at the measuring point closest to the site of
stimulation; a little later an action potential also appears at the second
measuring point. This shows that the action potential is *propagated* or
conducted from the site of stimulation past the first and second electrodes.

The *velocity of conduction* can be determined by dividing the
distance between the two measuring points that the action potential
passes by the time the action potential takes to travel between these
points. (A typical measurement of this sort could assume distance of
5 cm between the measuring points. If the traveling time between the
points is 2.5 msec, then the velocity of conduction is 0.05 m/0.0025 sec
= 20 m/sec.) The conduction velocities measured in nerve fibers
range from 1 m/sec to more than 100 m/sec. The conduction velocity
depends on the characteristics of the nerve fiber and is typical for each
type of fiber (see page 62).

Mechanism of propagation. It is characteristic of action potential conduction that the action potential signal is not weakened by this process. Therefore conduction *cannot take place solely* as a result of current flow from an excited to a nonexcited site. Such electrotonic transmission would generate potentials that became smaller with increasing distance from the site of current application. Instead, the amplitude of the action potential remains constant along the propagation path because an *excitation* occurs at every point on the membrane. These local responses obey the all-or-nothing law.

Electrotonic transmission and excitation act together in the conduction of the action potential. Current flows from an already excited point on the membrane to a neighboring and as yet unexcited, undepolarized region, where it generates an *electrotonic potential*. This potential reaches the threshold and serves as the *stimulus* initiating excitation in this part of the membrane. The process of excitation now takes place automatically at this point and in turn supplies current for the electrotonic depolarization of other regions of the membrane.

The action potential is conducted like the spark in a blasting fuse. At the point where the fuse is lit the gunpowder explodes (excitation); as a result the neighboring section of the fuse is warmed (electrotonic potential) to the point where the gunpowder there also explodes and in turn supplies heat for igniting the next sections.

Membrane currents during a propagated action potential. Figure 2-21 illustrates in detail the relationships between membrane voltage and membrane currents when an action potential is propagated. The figure represents an "action shot" of the voltage and current conditions along the fiber. The action potential is being conducted from right to left. The total length of the fiber covered by the action potential depends on the velocity of conduction. Given a fiber conducting at a velocity of 100 m/sec and an action potential of 1 msec duration, the length of the abscissa in Fig. 2-21 would correspond to 10 cm. Since the action potential travels past a particular point on the membrane at the conduction velocity, Fig. 2-21 can also be seen as representing the time course of the action potential at one point on the fiber. The abscissa would then, for example, be 1 msec long.

The action potential and below it the conductance curves g_K *and* g_{Na} have already been illustrated in Fig. 2-16 where the changes in conductance during the action potential were discussed (see page 46). As a result of the change in g_{Na} and g_K, sodium and potassium currents flow. The sum of these currents is shown under the conductance curves in Fig. 2-21 as the total ionic current, i_i.

The charge transported through the membrane by the ionic current i_i can follow two different paths: first, it can flow locally into the

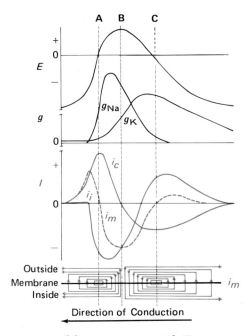

Fig. 2-21. Propagation of the action potential. Topmost curve: time course of, or local change in, action potential along the fiber. Below that, the membrane conductances g_{Na} and g_K (see Fig. 2-6). Below these, the membrane current components: ionic current, i_i, capacitative current, i_c, and the membrane current i_m. The broken vertical lines are drawn at A, the point of steepest slope, B, the maximum values of the action potential, and C the point of maximum repolarization velocity. (From Noble: *Physiol. Rev.* **46**, 1, 1966.)

membrane capacity, thereby discharging it. This current component is plotted alongside the ionic current i_i in Fig. 2-21 and is called *capacitative current, i_c.* Second, it can flow through the membrane via the membrane resistance. In elongated cells this current flows for a certain distance along the fiber because of the potential differences along the latter, for example, between excited and unexcited points. This current component, i_m, is also plotted in Fig. 2-21 together with the total ionic current i_i. The current lines of the *membrane current, i_m,* are depicted diagrammatically in the lower part of Fig. 2-21.

The amplitude of the capacitative current i_c at any point on the membrane is proportional to the change in potential at this point (see page 49). The amplitude of the membrane current in any region of the membrane is proportional to the membrane conductance and the displacement of the membrane potential from the relevant equilibrium potential. The density of the membrane current along the fiber is proportional to the potential differences along the fiber.

We must now discuss the behavior of the various current components during the course of the propagated action potential. As can be seen from Fig. 2-21, at the start of the propagated action potential there is still no appreciable ionic current i_i during the initial *slow rising phase*. In this phase the membrane is *depolarized* by the *outflowing membrane current i_m*, which entered the fiber at the adjacent excited region (to the right of the vertical line A). The threshold range is reached as a result of this electrotonic depolarization of the membrane. When this happens, and not before, g_{Na} increases, and the Na^+ influx sets up a negative ionic current i_i. At first i_i remains smaller than the capacitative current i_c because, up to the steepest part of the action potential (vertical line A), membrane current from the adjacent, fully excited region still helps to discharge the membrane capacity.

In the *second part of the upstroke* of the action potential, between A and B, i_c is smaller than i_i. More current is flowing in than is needed to discharge the membrane capacity. The excess flows as membrane current i_m through the membrane and on through the inside of the fiber where it serves to *depolarize adjacent membrane regions*. Finally, at the *peak* of the action potential the total ionic current i_i flows as i_m through the membrane. At the peak of the propagated action potential the sodium influx is therefore still considerably larger than the potassium efflux. The difference is used to drive still unexcited regions to the threshold "in front of" the action potential by means of membrane current.

After the peak of the action potential the negative ionic current i_i decreases rapidly, since g_{Na} falls and g_K rises. A lot of current flows from the region with positive potentials into the adjacent regions. i_i becomes smaller than i_m, the membrane potential must fall, and *repolarization* is initiated. Finally, the positive potassium efflux predominates, and the net ionic current i_i becomes positive. At C the current i_i is of the same magnitude as the current i_c, which restores the negative membrane charge. In the last phase of the propagated action potential, beyond C, the repolarization is again slowed down by current flow i_m from the fully excited region. In this phase, i_m depolarizes the membrane just as it did at the start of the action potential (left of A). This depolarizing membrane current is, however, more than compensated for by *potassium outflow* at high g_K.

If the potassium outflow at the end of repolarization is no longer sufficient to compensate for the depolarizing membrane current i_m, the membrane can be depolarized to the threshold again after almost complete repolarization, and further excitation can follow. Such *repetitive excitations* can easily be triggered if i_m is supported by a lasting depolarizing current flow from another current source, for example, an excitatory synapse or a receptor (see page 193).

The following current components thus predominate during the various *phases* of the propagated action potential. During the first half of the upstroke, membrane current flows as electrotonic current from the adjacent already excited region of the membrane and depolarizes the membrane to the threshold. Around the peak of the action potential, predominantly Na^+ current flows into the fiber. The greater part of this current flows as membrane current into adjacent regions of the fiber. During the second half of the repolarization process, chiefly K^+ current flows out of the fiber. This recharges the membrane to the resting value and counteracts the depolarizing membrane current that is generated in the excited region.

The *time course* of the capacitative current i_c and the membrane current i_m can be described in very simple mathematical terms. i_c is proportional to the first derivative of the time course of the membrane potential (see page 49). i_m corresponds to the change of i_c along the fiber and hence the change with time. i_m is therefore proportional to the second derivative of the membrane potential with respect to time. During an action potential an electrode placed on the outside of a nerve fiber measures voltage changes proportional to i_m in the surrounding bathing solution. Such *extracellular recordings* of an action potential have the same triphasic time course as i_m in Fig. 2-21. The extracellularly recorded potential is first positive, then strongly negative, and then positive again.

Factors affecting the velocity of conduction; saltatory conduction.
The velocity of conduction of the action potential can be calculated, with a great deal of effort, from the potential and the time dependence of the ionic currents as well as from the parameters fiber diameter, membrane capacity, and membrane resistance, which determine the spread of electrotonic potentials. At this point we shall deal only qualitatively with the factors influencing the velocity of propagation.

The velocity of conduction increases with the *amplitude of the Na*$^+$ *influx*, because if more current is available during excitation following discharge of the membrane capacity, then more current can flow into and accelerate the depolarization of adjacent, still unexcited regions. When an excitation starts from a normal resting potential the Na^+ influx into the cell is at its maximum level, and as a result the maximum velocity of conduction is also attained. If the resting potential is lowered (that is, becomes less negative) the Na^+ system is partially inactivated, and the Na^+ influx is reduced during excitation (see page 45). Therefore, *when the resting potential is lowered, the velocity of conduction is reduced.*

In addition, the *electrotonic flow* of the membrane currents has an important effect on the velocity of conduction. If the electrotonic potentials rise faster and if they decline less with distance, the conduction velocity must increase. The electrotonic potential will rise faster if the membrane capacity is reduced, and it will fall less with distance if the membrane resistance is increased. These conditions are utilized in the *medullated nerves* to increase the velocity of conduction. In these nerve fibers the membrane is thickened by the buildup of insulating myelin layers (see page 8) that greatly increases its resistance. In the medullated parts of these nerve fibers, the internodes, an electrotonic potential declines only slightly with distance. The action potential is therefore *propagated over the internodes at very high speed.*

If the propagated action potentials illustrated in Fig. 2-22 are measured simultaneously at many points on a medullated nerve, it is found that the action potential is not measurably retarded in the individual internodes (thick sections of nerve in Fig. 2-22). On the other hand, propagation is retarded at the *nodes of Ranvier R_1-R_5.* There is no myelin sheath at these nodes, and consequently the membrane capacity and resistance are normal. At these points the electrotonic potential increases slowly, and the excitation starts with a delay which is apparent at each node in Fig. 2-22. In medullated nerve fibers the excitation jumps from node to node, and the conduction of the excitation is therefore called "saltatory." Since the propaga-

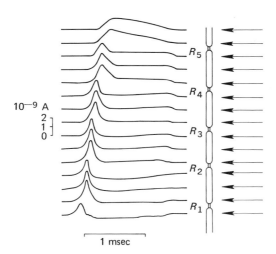

Fig. 2-22. Saltatory conduction of excitation. Left: Time courses of the membrane potential measured at the points indicated by the arrows (right) on a medullated axon. R_1, R_2, R_3 . . . are the nodes of Ranvier. The conduction of the action potential (from bottom to top) is delayed at each of the nodes. (From Huxley and Stämpfli: *J. Physiol.* **108**, 1, 1949.)

tion time between the nodes is so short, the overall velocity of propagation is much higher in medullated fibers than in nonmedullated fibers of the same thickness. In vertebrates, all the fibers that conduct at velocities of propagation in excess of 3 m/sec are medullated.

Along with myelination, which increases the velocity of conduction, the *fiber diameter* is the other most important factor determining the propagation velocity. The resistance to the passage of current along the fiber decreases with the square of the inside fiber diameter. When the *resistance along the fiber is low*, relatively more current flows from the excited region to the adjacent regions, which are then more rapidly depolarized by electrotonic current. Thus the velocity of propagation rises with the increase in fiber diameter.

The dependence of the velocity of conduction on the fiber diameter is shown in Table 2-2 for afferent (sensory) nerves of warm-blooded animals. The nerve fibers are categorized according to a generally accepted scheme into Groups I to IV. The nerve fibers of Groups I to III are medullated; those of Group IV are unmedullated. The latter are frequently called C fibers (see also Table 1-1).

In the medullated fibers of Groups I to III the velocity of conduction increases at a faster rate than in proportion to the increase in fiber diameter. The unmedullated fibers of Group IV have very low speeds of conduction. If the speed of conduction of unmedullated fibers of varying thickness is also determined, it is found that here, too, the speed of conduction is higher with increasing fiber diameter. Extremely thick unmedullated fibers such as, for example, the giant axon of squid, which is 0.7 mm in diameter, have a speed of conduction in the region of 25 m/sec.

Mixed nerves at the periphery of the body, for example, the Nervus ischiaticus, which serves the musculature and the skin of the leg, contain all the fibers of Groups I to IV as well as efferent, chiefly motor, fibers. If such a nerve is stimulated at one end, the excitation is propagated at very different speeds in the various groups of fibers. If the action potential is measured at some distance from the site of

Table 2-2.   Groups of Fibers in Afferent Nerves of Cats.

Group	Examples of Their Function	Mean Fiber Diameter (μ)	Mean Conduction Velocity (m/sec)
I	Primary muscle spindle afferents	13	75
II	Mechanoreceptors of the skin	9	55
III	Deep pressure sensitivity of the muscle	3	11
IV	Unmedullated pain fibers	1	1

stimulation, the first action potential to arrive will be that of the fastest group of fibers, Group I. Next will come the slower action potential of the Group II fibers, and then that of the Group III fibers, finally followed by that of the Group IV fibers. Thus a spectrum of action potentials is generated after a stimulus. Given a conduction path of 1 m, and using the values listed in Table 2-2, the action potentials of Group I fibers would be recorded after 13 msec and those of Group IV fibers after 1 sec.

Answer the following questions to check your knowledge:

Q 2.22 Plot the course of the current lines (i_m) in an elongated cell from an excited region to adjacent regions. Beneath this, plot the time course of the action potential.

Q 2.23 Which is the source of the current that depolarizes the membrane to the threshold in a still unexcited area when the action potential is propagated?
a. The driving force for the potassium ions.
b. The sodium inflow of the still unexcited area of the membrane.
c. The sodium inflow of an adjacent, already excited part of the membrane.
d. The axoplasm of the cell.

Q 2.24 Which of the following statements applies to the current flow at the moment when the peak of the propagated action potential is reached? You may use Fig. 2-21 to help you solve this problem.
a. The Na^+ inflow is equal to the K^+ outflow.
b. The Na^+ inflow outweighs the K^+ outflow; the net current reverses the charge of the membrane capacity.
c. The Na^+ inflow outweighs the K^+ outflow; the net current flows into neighboring regions of the membrane and depolarizes them.
d. The K^+ outflow outweighs the Na^+ inflow; the net current depolarizes neighboring regions of the membrane.
e. At the peak of the action potential, no current flows into the membrane capacity.

Q 2.25 Which of the following factors reduces the velocity of conduction of a nerve?
a. Reduction in fiber diameter.
b. Decrease in resting potential by 10 mV.
c. Loss of the myelin sheath (in the event of degeneration).
d. Increase in the extracellular Na^+ concentration.
e. 50% reduction in the extracellular K^+ concentration.

3

SYNAPTIC TRANSMISSION

The junction of an axonal ending with a nerve cell, a muscle cell, or a glandular cell was first called a *synapse* by Sherrington (see also Chapter 1, page 3). At synapses the propagated action potential is transmitted to the next cell. Originally it was wrongly believed that the axon always formed a "tight junction," that is, was fused with the cell on which it ended so that the propagated impulse could be transmitted without interruption to this cell. However, electrophysiological and histological investigations have shown that this form of synapse, which is now called an *electrical synapse*, is rare. Another type of synapse is far commoner, particularly in mammals and thus in man. In this type, the axonal ending when stimulated releases a chemical substance that produces an excitatory or an inhibitory effect at the neighboring cell membrane. This type of synapse is called a *chemical synapse*. The structure and the function of excitatory and inhibitory chemical synapses will be explained in this chapter.

3.1 The Neuromuscular Junction: Example of a Chemical Synapse

Structural elements of chemical synapses. Light and electron microscope investigations have shown that synaptic junctions widely vary in shape and form. As regards function, however, all the parts of a chemical synapse can be related to the basic elements illustrated in Fig. 3-1 and discussed and described in the following paragraphs. In Fig. 3-1 the axon ends in the *presynaptic terminal*. Under the microscope this often stands out as a spherical enlargement of the end of the axon (cf. Fig. 3-9), called the "synaptic knob." The presynaptic terminal is separated from the postsynaptic side by a narrow cleft (gap), which is, on the average, 100 to 200 Å wide. This is known as the

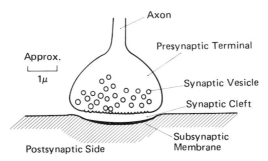

Fig. 3-1. Diagrammatic section through a chemical synapse. All the structural elements important for synaptic transmission are shown. The diameter of the synaptic vesicles is drawn disproportionately large relative to the other parts of the synapse.

synaptic cleft. It is clearly discernible only under the electron microscope. The postsynaptic membrane, which is located exactly opposite the presynaptic terminal forming the postsynaptic boundary of the synaptic cleft, is called the *subsynaptic membrane.* Under the electron microscope the subsynaptic membrane usually appears somewhat thicker than the other parts of the postsynaptic membrane, which indicates that is has a function different from that of the rest of the postsynaptic membrane.

The presynaptic terminal contains a large number of submicroscopic spherical structures that can be detected only under the electron microscope, namely, the *synaptic vesicles.* They are about 500 Å in diameter. Many experimental findings, the most important of which are discussed in this chapter, indicate that the synaptic vesicles in the presynaptic terminals contain the *transmitter substance* that is released into the synaptic cleft upon excitation and then triggers excitation or inhibition of the subsynaptic membrane.

The motoaxons of the motoneurons in the ventral horn of the spinal cord form synapses with striated muscle fibers (skeletal muscle fibers). Because of its appearance, this synapse, and, in particular, the presynaptic section, is called the *neuromuscular end plate* or, alternatively, the *neuromuscular junction* (Fig. 3-2). It possesses all the typical morphological characteristics of a chemical synapse; that is, in addition to the presynaptic terminal with its characteristic synaptic vesicles, it has a synaptic cleft and a subsynaptic membrane on the postsynaptic side. However, in this case, instead of being a nerve cell the postsynaptic side consists of a skeletal muscle fiber. It is possible to remove such muscles, together with the associated nerves, from the living organism and to place them in a blood-substitute solution (for example, Ringer solution or Tyrode solution) where they remain alive

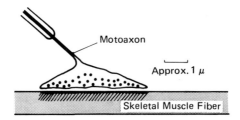

Fig. 3-2. Diagrammatic section through a neuromuscular junction (end plate). The synaptic vesicles are not drawn on the same scale as the rest of the synapse; they appear larger here than they really are. Only part of a skeletal muscle fiber is shown.

and functioning for some time. The Musculus gastrocnemius and the M. sartorius, with the associated nerves of the same name, from frogs, and the diaphragm, plus the Nervus phrenicus from rats, are well-known preparations of this type.

Detection of the end-plate potential. Figure 3-3 illustrates the experimental setup for studying synaptic transmission at the neuro-muscular junction of an *in vitro* preparation of a skeletal muscle. The figure shows a muscle fiber with its motoaxon. A microelectrode is inserted into the muscle fiber to record its membrane potential intra-cellularly. As soon as this microelectrode is advanced from the bath-ing solution into the interior of the muscle cell, a resting potential of about −70 mV is indicated on a cathode-ray oscilloscope or some other suitable measuring instrument (Fig. 3-4). If the associated moto-axon is now stimulated electrically, an action potential propagates down into the presynaptic terminal of the end plate. On the postsyn-

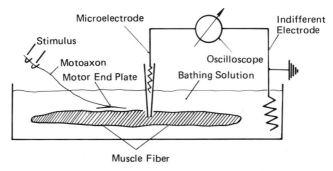

Fig. 3-3. Experimental arrangement for recording end-plate potentials. The intracellular microelectrode records the changes in potential at the mus-cle fiber membrane relative to the external bath electrode. The motoaxon is electrically stimulated. To prevent short-circuiting between the stimulating electrodes, the nerve is held in air or under a film of paraffin oil during stimulation.

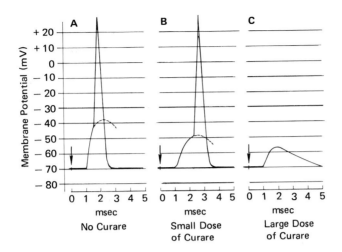

Fig. 3-4. End-plate potentials recorded by an intracellular microelectrode. Experimental arrangement as in Fig. 3-3. A: Changes in intracellular potential following stimulation of the associated motoaxon. Muscle fiber in normal Ringer solution. B: Small amount of curare added to the bathing solution. C: Curare concentration doubled.

aptic side, that is, at the membrane of the muscle fiber, it triggers the potential changes indicated in Fig. 3-4A. The arrow in Fig. 3-4A denotes the moment at which the stimulus was applied to the moto-axon. After a latent period of about 1 msec (depending on the length of the nerve and the conduction velocity of the motoaxon), the muscle membrane potential depolarizes to the threshold, and a typical action potential appears (cf. Figs. 2-10 and 2-11). It can be seen clearly how the initial depolarization converts into the steep upstroke of the action potential at about − 42 mV. The propagated action potential makes the muscle fiber contract (for details, see Chapter 5).

If a small quantity (10^{-7} to 10^{-6} g/ml) of the poison curare is added to the bathing solution, and if the motoaxon is again stimulated, the changes in membrane potential shown in Fig. 3-4B are recorded. The initial depolarization is slower, and therefore the action potential starts a little later. However, the pattern of the action potential remains unchanged, and a muscular contraction is still observed. But, if still more curare is added to the bathing solution (Fig. 3-4C), the initial depolarization no longer evokes an action potential; instead, it remains subthreshold and returns to the resting potential after a few milliseconds. (The muscle does not contract either.) The potential remaining after the action potential disappears is called the *end-plate potential (EPP)*. The dotted lines in Fig. 3-4A and B indicate the time courses of EPPs masked by the superimposed action potentials. End-plate potentials can thus vary in amplitude, being either suprathreshold or subthreshold.

In healthy muscles the EPPs are always far above threshold. Each presynaptic action potential triggers a contraction in the associated muscle fibers. The amplitude of the normally suprathreshold end-plate potential is severely reduced by poisoning with curare, and if the curare concentration is high enough, the EPP falls below the threshold. That is, it no longer triggers any action potential in the muscle fiber nor any contraction. Neuromuscular transmission is therefore *blocked* by curare. Thus a person poisoned by curare will asphyxiate because neuromuscular transmission in his striated muscles, and these include his respiratory muscles, is blocked.

The experiment just described and illustrated in Figs. 3-3 and 3-4 is not by itself enough to permit conclusions regarding what presynaptic and postsynaptic events lead to the generation of the EPP or how curare, for example, reduces the amplitude of the EPP. Intensive experimental analysis extending back several decades, and still going on in some areas, was necessary to clarify these relationships. The results obtained will be summarized in the following paragraph, and then the most important facts will be dealt with in more detail.

The action potential invading the presynaptic terminal releases a certain amount of transmitter substance into the synaptic cleft. The transmitter substances diffuses to the subsynaptic membrane and induces permeability changes that lead to the generation of the EPP. The transmitter substance at the neuromuscular junction is acetylcholine. It acts on the subsynaptic membrane for only a very short time because it is broken down by an enzyme, cholinesterase, into two inactive components, choline and acetic acid.

Even this very brief description shows that there are a number of ways in which the transmission at a chemical synapse may be influenced. A drug, for example, may inhibit synaptic transmission by preventing impulse propagation into the presynaptic ending; by blocking the mechanism that releases transmitter substance when an action potential invades the presynaptic terminal; by inhibiting the production or storage of the transmitter substance; by combining with the transmitter substance at the synaptic cleft to form an inactive compound; or by quickly breaking down the transmitter substance into inactive components. Finally, it may compete with the transmitter substance for the receptor sites on the subsynaptic membrane. Examples can be given for almost all of these possibilities. Curare, for instance, *competes* with ACh for its receptors at the subsynaptic membrane.

The nature of the end-plate potential. In the following we will consider which changes in the subsynaptic membrane lead to the generation of the EPP. We will first see that the EPP is generated only at the subsynaptic membrane. Then some experiments will be described which prove that the EPP is the result of a brief increase in the permeability of the membrane to small cations (Na$^+$, K$^+$, Ca^{++}).

Figure 3-5 shows the intracellular recording of an EPP at various distances from the end plate in a nerve-muscle preparation treated with curare. The impalements are spaced about 1 mm apart. It is apparent that as the microelectrode is inserted further away from the end plate, the amplitude of the EPP decreases, and its rise and decay times become longer. This finding is a clear indication of the passive electrotonic spreading of the EPP from its site of generation, the subsynaptic membrane (see Sec. 2.6). Thus it can be stated that excitation of the end plate at the subsynaptic membrane gives rise to a depolarization, the end-plate potential. Provided it remains below the threshold (that is, does not trigger a propagated action potential), this EPP spreads electrotonically along the muscle fiber in accordance with the passive electrical characteristics of the muscle fiber membrane.

Voltage clamp tests and mathematical analysis of the time course and the spatial distribution of the EPP lead to the conclusion that the initial phase of depolarization, which occurs while the transmitter substance acetylcholine (ACh) reacts with the subsynaptic membrane, lasts only about 1 to 2 msec. In other words, the change in membrane permeability that leads to a shift in charge at the membrane capacitor takes place in this short time. The subsequent time course of the EPP is determined by the passive electrical characteristics of the muscle fiber membrane, that is, by the membrane capacity and resistance.

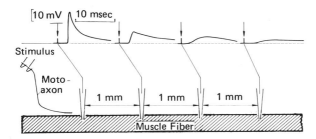

Fig. 3-5. Electrotonic nature of the end-plate potential. EPP recorded with an intracellular microelectrode. Experimental arrangement as in Fig. 3-3. Sufficient curare is added to the bathing solution to prevent the generation of action potentials in the muscle fiber when the associated motoaxon is stimulated. EPP recorded at increasing distance from the end plate.

The nature of the changes in permeability during the initial phase of the EPP was revealed most clearly by determining the equilibrium potential of the EPP in normal bathing solution and then after systematic variation of the extracellular ionic concentration. An experimental setup for measuring the equilibrium potential of the EPP—the membrane potential at which no change in potential occurs during the action of ACh—is sketched in Fig. 3-6. In addition to the recording electrode, a second microelectrode is inserted into the muscle fiber. This second electrode is connected to a current source, enabling the membrane potential to be varied at will.

The right half of Fig. 3-6 shows the effect of the stimulus at four different membrane potentials with the muscle fiber held in normal bathing solution. If the EPP is evoked at a membrane potential of -95 mV, its amplitude is approximately 15 mV in the depolarizing direction; at -45 mV the amplitude is 5 mV in the depolarizing direction; at -15 mV the amplitude is 0 mV, and at $+30$ mV it is 15 mV in the hyperpolarizing direction. This result shows that under normal conditions the equilibrium potential of the EPP (E_{EPP}) is located approximately at -15 mV, that is, between the equilibrium potentials for potassium ($E_K = -80$ mV) and sodium ($E_{Na} = +45$ mV).

These and other measurements lead to the conclusion that during the time that the ACh acts on the subsynaptic membrane, for about 1 to 2 msec, *the permeability of the membrane to small cations (Na$^+$, K$^+$) is increased considerably.* Under normal circumstances, there-

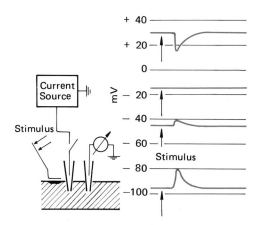

Fig. 3-6. The equilibrium potential of the EPP. The experimental setup is sketched on the left. It corresponds to that in Fig. 3-3. A second microelectrode is inserted in the fiber for the application of current from an external source to vary the membrane potential of the muscle fiber. The arrows in the right half of the figure indicate the suprathreshold stimulation of the associated motoaxon.

fore, the given ionic distribution (see Table 2-1) will result in predominantly Na^+ ions flowing into the muscle fiber. This reduces the membrane potential, because at a membrane potential of -70 mV the driving force for the Na^+ ions is more powerful than that for the K^+ ions; there is a net inward current carried by Na^+ ions. If the change in permeability is large enough, the muscle fiber membrane at the end plate is depolarized to the threshold, and a propagated action potential which spreads out over the entire fiber membrane is evoked (see Fig. 3-4). Pharmacological experiments indicate that separate pores or channels for Na^+ and K^+ exist at the subsynaptic membrane. Procaine, for instance, influences the time course of the change in Na^+ conductance, but that for K^+ remains unaffected.

The fate of the acetylcholine. Normally, after its release from the presynaptic terminal, the ACh diffuses across the synaptic cleft to the subsynaptic membrane where it combines with *receptors*. The ACh takes only fractions of a millisecond to diffuse across the narrow synaptic cleft. It combines with the subsynaptic receptors and causes an increase in the membrane permeability for small cations.

To use a metaphor, the AC*h* key is inserted in the *receptor* lock, and the *permeability* door *for small cations is opened wide.* However, the ACh can act for only 1 to 2 msec at the subsynaptic membrane since, as already briefly mentioned, it is broken down by the enzyme cholinesterase into the inactive components choline and acetic acid. (Special staining methods have shown that cholinesterase is present in large quantities at the end plate. In addition, cholinesterase also circulates in the blood so that ACh that diffuses from an end plate into the surrounding extracellular space and thus into the circulation is also split into choline and acetic acid.) The decomposition products of ACh, choline and acetic acid, are for the most part reabsorbed by the presynaptic terminal and, with the aid of enzymes, resynthesized to ACh which is stored in the synaptic vesicles of the presynaptic terminal until it is released once more. This ACh cycle is shown diagrammatically in Fig. 3-7.

If ACh is applied electrophoretically to a muscle fiber with a micropipette, it evokes depolarizations only at the end plate but not in other sections of the muscle fiber membrane. It can be concluded that the ACh receptors are located only at the subsynaptic membrane and nowhere else on the postsynaptic membrane. Injection of ACh into the muscle fiber likewise fails to produce depolarization of the membrane because ACh, like all other transmitter substances, acts only on the outer surface of the subsynaptic membrane. (It is interesting to note that the sensitivity of the subsynaptic membrane to ACh spreads to the remainder of the muscle fiber in the event of degeneration of

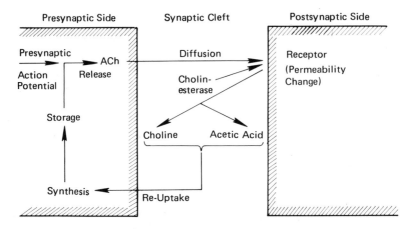

Fig. 3-7. Metabolic cycle of acetylcholine in the neuromuscular junction. See text for details.

the end plate following section of the presynaptic axon; this process is reversed when reinnervation occurs.)

Inhibition of the cholinesterase activity in the synaptic cleft results in a prolonged interaction of ACh with its subsynaptic receptors. The permeability of the subsynaptic membrane for small cations remains increased for a protracted period, and the EPP becomes larger and much longer. The E_{EPP} is located at approximately -15 mV, and if the inhibition of the cholinesterase activity is strong enough, the muscle fiber membrane adjacent to the end plate may depolarize to such an extent that the Na^+ transport mechanism is inactivated and the membrane becomes inexcitable. A large number of substances are known to have an inhibitory effect on cholinesterase, such as therapeutic drugs and insecticides. Poison gases (war gases) have also been developed that act in the same way.

Substances that block neuromuscular transmission are used during anesthesia to relax the muscles. A patient treated with this sort of drug requires artificial respiration, but the anesthesia need only be deep enough to render the person unconscious and eliminate the sensation of pain without suppressing motor reflexes. A shallow state of anesthesia has the advantage of being less toxic, easier to control, and quickly reversible. Substances that relax the muscles during anesthesia or in other therapeutic situations are called *muscle relaxants.*

Curare and similarly acting substances are muscle relaxants and are used in medical practice. However, these substances do not act by inhibiting the cholinesterase; instead, as already mentioned, they compete with the transmitter substance for its subsynaptic receptors. A second group of muscle relaxants, also used in practice, acts in yet another way: these substances, like ACh, act on the subsynaptic membrane, but they cannot be broken down or are broken down only very slowly by cholinesterase (for example, succinylcholine).

The different modes of action of the various muscle relaxants also can be used therapeutically. For example, the insecticide E 605 inhibits the cholinesterase in insects. After an intermediate stage of increased muscle excitability (cramp), it induces a state of respiratory paralysis and death. The effect is similar in humans if E 605 is ingested or administered. In these circumstances, the patient should be treated not only with E 605-deactivating substances but also with substances similar to curare that alleviate the blocking of neuromuscular transmission. Conversely, in the event of poisoning by curare, it is possible to increase the reduced and possibly subthreshold EPP and to restore normal neuromuscular transmission by inhibiting the cholinesterase activity. In the muscular disease myasthenia gravis pseudoparalytica, resynthesis of the ACh in the presynaptic terminal is slowed down so that if the synapse is repetitively activated there is a decrease in the amount of transmitted substance released. This finally leads to complete blocking of neuromuscular transmission. A typical symptom of this disease is that the patient's neuromuscular transmission is good in the morning but grows worse as the day progresses (drooping eyelids). Here, too, an effective and so far the only known method of treatment is to administer a cholinesterase inhibitor such as prostigmine. Thus, inhibition of the cholinesterase activity can promote or inhibit neuromuscular transmission, depending on the circumstances and also the degree of cholinesterase inhibition.

Answer the following questions to check your newly acquired knowledge.

Q 3.1 The EPP of a muscle fiber is generated by a brief increase in the permeability of the subsynaptic membrane for
    a. K^+ ions.
    b. Na^+ ions.
    c. Cl^- ions.
    d. ACh.
    e. Cholinesterase.
    f. Curare.

Q 3.2 Depolarization of a muscle fiber membrane to approximately -30 mV
    a. leaves the EPP unchanged.
    b. shortens the duration of the EPP considerably.
    c. increases the duration of the EPP considerably.
    d. prevents the generation of the EPP.
    e. none of the above is correct.

Q 3.3 Inhibition of cholinesterase blocks neuromuscular transmission
    because
    a. ACh is competitively driven away from its receptor.
    b. ACh is no longer released presynaptically.
    c. ACh is not broken down and consequently a lasting depolari-
       zation of the subsynaptic membrane occurs.
    d. the amplitude of the EPP is reduced to subthreshold values.
    e. none of the foregoing mechanisms applies.

Q 3.4 Which of the following statements are correct? In the event of
    poisoning by curare
    a. the presynaptic synthesis of ACh is not seriously affected.
    b. decomposition of the ACh after its release into the synaptic
       cleft is greatly slowed down.
    c. the ACh is competitively displaced from its subsynaptic re-
       ceptor.
    d. the equilibrium potential of the EPP shifts toward the resting
       potential.
    e. the time course of the EPP is considerably slowed down.

3.2   The Quantal Nature of Chemical Transmission

Miniature end-plate potentials and the quantum hypothesis. The
diagrams given in Figs. 3-1 and 3-2 showed that the presynaptic
terminal contains a large number of vesicles. It has already been
mentioned that these vesicles probably contain the transmitter substance. A few findings that support this assumption will now be discussed.

If a microelectrode is inserted into a *resting* muscle fiber (see
sketch in the bottom part of Fig. 3-8), small, brief, and irregularly
occurring depolarizations will be recorded (cf. Figs. 3-8A and B).
These spontaneous depolarizations are similar in their time course to
normal EPPs, but their amplitude is very much smaller than that of
normal EPPs (compare ordinate scale of Fig. 3-8 with that of Fig. 3-4).
Because of their similar time courses and very small amplitudes, these
spontaneous depolarizations are called *miniature end-plate potentials* (MEPPs). Experiments of the type illustrated in Fig. 3-5 have
shown clearly that the MEPPs, just as the EPPs, are generated only at
the subsynaptic membrane and spread out electrotonically from there
over the muscle fiber. (Because of their low amplitude they can only
be recorded in the direct vicinity of the end plate.) The pharmacological properties of the EPPs and the spontaneous MEPPs are also
identical. It is therefore justified to assume that the MEPPs are generated by the spontaneous release of small quantities of ACh.

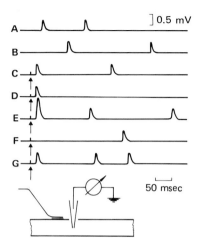

Fig. 3-8. Schematic representation of miniature end-plate potentials. Recording made with an intracellular microelectrode. Experimental arrangement as in Fig. 3-3. The Ca^{++} concentration in the bathing solution was reduced to 50% of normal and a few mMol of Mg^{++} ions were added. In traces C to G the associated motoaxon was stimulated electrically (arrows).

Figure 3-8 also shows that the MEPPs all have approximately the same amplitude. From this it may be concluded that they are triggered by approximately equal quantities of ACh. These nearly equal-sized packets of ACh are called *quanta*. By applying an experimental trick, it is possible to show that the normal EPP is also caused by the release of quanta of transmitter substance. The quantity of transmitter substance released per action potential may be reduced substantially by removing Ca^{++} ions from the bathing solution or by adding Mg^{++} ions. Records of EPPs triggered under these conditions are shown on the left in Fig. 3-8C–G. (In addition, some later occurring spontaneous MEPPs are seen.) A total of five stimuli (arrows) were applied. In C, D, and G the EPP was approximately as large as the spontaneous MEPPs; after the stimulus in E the EPP was about twice as large as the MEPPs, and following the stimulus F no EPP was seen. This finding suggests that the normal EPP also may always be composed of multiples of MEPPs; that is, it is caused by the simultaneous release of a large number of quanta.

This view has been confirmed in a large number of experiments. We may summarize the results as follows: at rest, the end plate releases single quanta of transmitter substance at irregular intervals (average frequency 1/sec). Each quantum triggers a MEPP at the subsynaptic membrane. In other words, there is a certain probability that at any given moment a quantum of transmitter substance will be released by the presynaptic terminal. During the presynaptic action potential the probability of quantal release is increased considerably for a very short time, so that within less than 1 msec several hundred quanta are released, triggering the normal EPP. It has been estimated that about 200 quanta per presynaptic action potential are released at the end plate in frog. In other synapses the release of transmitter substance is as high as 2000 quanta. The total amount of acetylcholine released at the end plate as the result of an action potential has been estimated to be 1.5×10^{-15} g.

If Ca^{++} ions are withdrawn from the bathing solution, the presynaptic action potential releases not several hundred but fewer quanta. The number of quanta released per pulse fluctuates around a mean value which depends on the effective Ca^{++} concentration. At low Ca^{++} concentrations EPPs appear whose amplitudes are low multiples of the MEPPs (see Fig. 3-8), and occasionally no quantum of transmitter is released. The size of the quanta does not vary. The results leave no doubt that the presence of Ca^{++} ions is absolutely essential for the normal course of quantal release triggered by a presynaptic action potential. The mechanism of Ca^{++} action is still unknown. Adding Mg^{++} ions has an effect similar to withdrawing Ca^{++} ions. Presumably, the Mg^{++} ions compete with the Ca^{++} ions for their sites of action at the presynaptic membrane. Four Ca^{++} ions seem to be needed for the release of one quantum of transmitter substance because the number of ACh quanta released depends approximately on the fourth power of the extracellular Ca^{++} concentration.

Neuromuscular blocking brought about by removing Ca^{++} or adding Mg^{++} cannot be used in humans, unlike the previously mentioned methods, because the functions of other organ systems, such as heart, kidney, CNS, and smooth muscles, are severely disrupted by these changes in the ionic medium. The toxin of botulinus bacteria (in spoiled foods) has an effect on the end plate similar to Ca^{++} removal. By inhibiting the release of ACh, botulinus toxin poisoning causes paralysis of the muscles, often fatal because it prevents respiration. Since botulinus toxin is sensitive to heat, an effective protection against poisoning is to boil or to fry the suspected foodstuff.

The "quantum hypothesis" rests basically on two findings: (1) the electron microscope discovery of the synaptic vesicles and (2) the physiological findings of the quantal nature of transmitter release. In the meantime, vesicles and MEPPs have been found in many other chemical synapses. It is also possible to isolate synaptic vesicles by ultracentrifugation. These vesicles were found to contain ACh or similar substances to which a transmitter function is ascribed. It is possible that quanta of transmitter substance are released at all these synapses, even at those whose transmitter has not yet been identified. Such a quantum (not to be confused with the energy quanta of physics) probably contains several thousand transmitter molecules that are discharged within a very short time into the very narrow ($< 0.1 \mu$) synaptic cleft and act practically simultaneously on the subsynaptic membrane. At a frog end plate a quantum contains about 10^3 to 10^4 ACh molecules, but no estimates are available for the other synapses. At present, it is not possible to ascribe any physiological function to the MEPPs.

Control of transmitter release by the presynaptic action potential. Increasing the extracellular K^+ concentration lowers the membrane potential (see page 24). At the same time, in a preparation such as that illustrated in Fig. 3-8, it is observed that an increase in the extracellular K^+ concentration increases the frequency of the MEPPs. Also, when the presynaptic membrane potential is lowered by applying current from an external source, the frequency of the MEPPs increases. These results indicate that the probability of quantal release depends at least in part on the membrane potential of the presynaptic terminal: the frequency of the MEPPs increases when the membrane potential is depolarized, and vice versa.

The action potential is a large, if only brief, depolarization of the membrane potential. Nevertheless, it seems capable of increasing the probability of transmitter release many thousand times above the resting value for a period of less than 1 msec, resulting in the sudden release of several hundred quanta of transmitter. More experimental data are needed to support this hypothesis, but a number of experiments, in particular varying the action potential amplitude by changing the resting potential and simulation of action potentials with current pulses applied through extracellular micropipettes, have provided good evidence that the magnitude of the EPP, that is, the number of quanta released per action potential, is dependent on the amplitude of this action potential.

Apart from this, unfortunately, we know very little about the events occurring between the arrival of the action potential in the presynaptic terminal and the start of the postsynaptic potential. This is a pity, because the synapse is possibly one of the most important substrates of the plasticity of the brain (learning, memory, and so on). For example, if the presynaptic resting potential is increased by frequent use of the synapse, each subsequent action potential will also be increased in amplitude, and as a result the synaptic transmission will be improved: the synapse is facilitated (posttetanic potentiation, see page 100). In addition, one can imagine that frequent use may lead to an extension of the synaptic contact area, stimulate the synthesis of transmitter substance, or result in increased availability of transmitter substance at the synaptic cleft (mobilization)—all of which should improve the synaptic transmission. In this way frequently used reflexes could be "learned" while others could be "forgotten" by reverse processes. Only when these relations are fully understood can we try to influence them specifically. That is, to facilitate or to inhibit synaptic transmission at certain synapses, for example, by pharmacological means, in order to influence the learning process or memory.

The importance of Ca^{++} for the release of transmitter substance has already been pointed out. Rather than at the end plate the role of Ca^{++} has been studied in greater detail at giant synapses in squid. The following results were obtained: depolarization of the presynaptic membrane potential either by an action potential or by a current pulse opens the "Ca^{++} pores" of the presynaptic membrane. This process has a threshold at 30 to 40 mV depolarization, and the extent of the Ca^{++} permeability change depends on the magnitude and the duration of the depolarization. The amount of transmitter substance released increases corresponding to the magnitude and the duration of the depolarization. Just as at the end plate, Mg^{++} and also Mn^{++} prevent the action of Ca^{++} at the presynaptic terminal, and thus also prevent the transmitter release. Ca^{++} is also required at other peripheral synapses for normal release of the transmitter substance; therefore it must be assumed that it plays the same role at all chemical synapses.

Answer the following questions to check your knowledge.

Q 3.5 Which of the following statements regarding MEPPs are correct?
   a. MEPPs are caused by the release of *one* molecule of ACh.
   b. The frequency of MEPPs is independent of the membrane potential of the presynaptic terminal.
   c. The time course of MEPPs is similar to that of normal EPPs.
   d. Curare reduces the amplitude of MEPPs or renders them completely undetectable.
   e. Cholinesterase inhibitors do not affect MEPPs.
   f. MEPPs improve synaptic transmission.

Q 3.6 Which of the following factors *increases* the number of quanta of transmitter substance released per presynaptic action potential?
   a. Decrease in the Ca^{++} concentration in the bathing solution.
   b. Addition of cholinesterase inhibitors to the bathing solution.
   c. Increase in the amplitude of the presynaptic action potential.
   d. Addition of curare to the bathing solution.
   e. Decrease in the Mg^{++} concentration in the bathing solution.

Q 3.7 Which of the following findings at the end plate supports the hypothesis that the presynaptic vesicles contain the transmitter substance?
  a. The presence of Ca^{++} is necessary for the release of ACh.
  b. MEPPs occur at the end plate.
  c. MEPPs are generated in a random sequence.
  d. The transmitter substance is always released in multiples of a mininum amount.
  e. Decrease in the presynaptic resting potential increases the frequency of the MEPPs.

3.3 Central Excitatory Synapses

With the neuromuscular junction as an example, we have learned the basic events that take place during the activation of a chemical synapse. We are now in a position to examine the somewhat more complex events occurring during excitatory transmission at central neurons. While each muscle fiber possesses only one end plate, and while each EPP is normally far above the threshold, central neurons usually possess many dozen to several thousand synapses, and the excitatory postsynaptic potentials of individual synapses are almost always subthreshold; consequently, only the simultaneous activity of a large number of synapses can give rise to a propagated action potential. In addition to the excitatory synapses, there are inhibitory synapses on the soma and the dendrites of neurons. Activation of the inhibitory synapses impedes the generation of a propagated action potential.

The motoneurons in the ventral horn of the spinal cord gray matter, whose nerve fibers (motoaxons) leave the spinal cord through the ventral roots and innervate skeletal muscle fibers, have proved particularly suitable for the study of neuronal synaptic potentials. They are large (diameter of soma up to 100 μ), are relatively easily accessible, and their excitatory and inhibitory connections are well known. Moreover, the results obtained from the motoneurons also apply without any great reservations to the majority of other central neurons. Consequently, these results can form the basis of our discussion.

Excitatory postsynaptic potentials (EPSPs). Figure 3-9 shows diagrammatically that, with the exception of the axon hillock and the axon, a large number of synapses are distributed over the surface of a neuron. It is estimated that each motoneuron possesses a total of about 6,000 axosomatic and axodendritic synapses. Some of these synapses are excitatory and some are inhibitory. Their presynaptic axons stem,

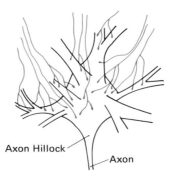

Axon Hillock

Axon

Fig. 3-9. Extremely simplified diagrammatic representation of motoneural synapses. The dendrites are cut off soon after their emergence from the soma. On this scale, they would extend far beyond the page of this book.

for the most part, from central neurons. However, some of the axons of excitatory synapses come directly from stretch receptors of the skeletal muscles, the muscle spindles; these axons are afferent nerve fibers which enter the spinal cord from the muscle nerves by the dorsal roots. As will be shown in detail later (Sec. 4.2) the muscle spindle afferents form direct excitatory synapses only with motoneurons of their own (homonymous) muscle. This situation makes it possible to activate excitatory synapses of a motoneuron by peripheral electric stimulation of the associated muscle. The postsynaptic processes can then be observed by means of an intracellular microelectrode.

Such an experimental arrangement is shown on the left in Fig. 3-10. A microelectrode is inserted into the soma of a motoneuron, and the associated muscle spindle afferents are placed on stimulating electrodes at the periphery. The microelectrode records a resting potential of -70 mV. When the afferents are stimulated electrically (arrows in A, B, C) a depolarization of the membrane potential occurs after a short delay (latency). The time course of the depolarizations in Fig.

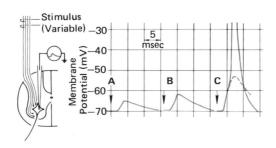

Fig. 3-10. Excitatory postsynaptic potentials. Intracellular recording from a motoneuron. Peripheral electrical stimulation of associated muscle nerve. Stimulus strength increases from A to C.

3-10A and B (not C!) is similar to that of the EPP. The amplitudes depend on the number of excited afferents, that is, on the strength of the stimulus in the case of electrical stimulation. The nerve was less strongly stimulated in A than in B. In C the nerve was stimulated even more strongly than in B, and the depolarization was so large that a propagated action potential occurred. Since the depolarizing potentials can excite the motoneuron, they are called *excitatory postsynaptic potentials (EPSPs)*.

The EPSPs are thus analogous to the EPPs at the neuromuscular junction. Whereas the EPP is generated by the activation of an individual synapse, namely, the neuromuscular junction, the EPSPs are usually caused by the simultaneous activation of several or many synapses. The rising phase of an EPSP lasts approximately 2 msec, and the decline lasts approximately 10 to 15 msec. As Figs. 3-10A and B show, the time course is independent of the amplitude of the EPSP. This means that the EPSPs elicited simultaneously at various synapses summate and do not influence each other's time course. (The unitary EPSPs are only independent of each other within certain limits, which need not be discussed here.)

In summary, stimulation of muscle spindle afferents generates an EPSP in motoneurons of the homonymous muscle. This EPSP possesses a typical and constant time course (rise time 2 msec, decay time 10 to 15 msec). The amplitude of the EPSP depends on the number of activated synapses. If this number is sufficiently large, the motoneuron is depolarized to the threshold and a propagated action potential occurs. (The latter runs via the motoaxon to the muscle and excites the muscle fibers which it innervates.)

Excitatory transmitter substances. Histologically, the synapses of the motoneurons are chemical synapses. The physiological characteristics of the EPSPs, such as the occurrence of miniature EPSPs, also indicate that the EPSPs are generated at the subsynaptic membrane through the action of a transmitter substance. Unfortunately, the chemical structure of the transmitter substance still has not been identified even though in recent years the suspicion has hardened that it is probably an amino acid. Nor do we know anything about the enzyme systems that inactivate the transmitter substance in the synaptic cleft and synthesize it in the presynaptic terminal.

Our knowledge of the synaptic transmitter substance or substances at most of the other excitatory synapses in the central nervous system is equally sketchy. This is an extremely unsatisfactory state of affairs, because, as was explained in the case of the end plate, the synapse offers a particularly large number of sites where pharmacological substances can act. We must assume that many drugs acting on the central nervous system have their action site at some link in the chain of chemical synaptic transmission. In view of these gaps in our knowledge, neurophysiologists and neuropharmacologists can at present give only sketchy details concerning the site and the mechanism of action of centrally acting drugs such as anesthetics, sedatives, psychopharmacological agents, and narcotics. Statements such as the following are made: "x increases the excitability of the Formatio reticularis," or "y has a sedative effect on the limbic system," or "z leads to a reduction in muscle tonus by inhibiting spinal interneurons." It is quite obvious that we cannot be content indefinitely with such vague and woolly statements.

The ionic mechanism of the EPSP and the triggering of the action potential.   Remember that the EPP is caused by a brief increase in permeability to small cations (Na^+, K^+). Since the EPSPs correspond in many respects to the EPPs, it is assumed that the EPSPs are also generated by a brief increase in permeability to small cations. (In addition, there also seems to be increased permeability to Cl^- ions.) This assumption is based, among other things, on the fact that the equilibrium potential of the EPSP is at approximately the same membrane potential as that of the EPP, that is, at approximately -15 mV. From the time course of the EPSP and the membrane time constant of the motoneurons, it was possible to calculate that the change in permeability for small cations lasts for about as long as the corresponding permeability change at the activated neuromuscular junction, namely 1 to 2 msec. The unknown transmitter substance thus acts for about the same time at the subsynaptic membrane of the motoneuron as the acetylcholine acts at the neuromuscular junction. (Many pharmacological tests have shown beyond all doubt that the transmitter substance of the motoneuronal EPSP is certainly not ACh.)

When the EPSPs are above the threshold, propagated action potentials are triggered (Fig. 3-10C). It has been found that the membrane of the motoneuron has its lowest threshold at the point where the axon leaves the soma, the *axon hillock* (see Fig. 3-9). The threshold of the soma and the dendrites is at least twice as high as that of the axon hillock. Propagated action potentials are therefore generated in motoneurons and probably also in other, if not all, nerve cells at the axon hillock. The advantage of the higher threshold of the soma and the dendrites compared with the axon hillock is that no matter which of the synapses are activated at any one time all the excitatory postsynaptic potentials have a common site of action, namely, the axon hillock. Since the axon hillock merges into the axon, this arrangement also guarantees that once an action potential has been evoked it will continue into the periphery, regardless of the conditions obtaining at the soma and the dendrites. Seen in this way, it is of no importance for the function of the nerve cells whether or not the action potential propagates into the soma and the dendrites.

Since the EPSPs are not actively propagated but spread out electrotonically on the cell membrane, one would expect that axo-somatic synapses in the vicinity of the axon hillock would have a greater influence on the excitability of a motoneuron than axo-somatic and axo-dendritic synapses located further away. This is perhaps in part correct. But this imbalance seems to be compensated for to some extent by the fact that particularly large EPSPs are generated at the dendrites. (This is probably not brought about by an increased release of transmitter substance but by the cable properties of the dendrites; that is, the cause is on the postsynaptic side.) The views of neurophysiologists on the relative importance of axo-somatic versus axo-dendritic synapses are, however, still very much at variance.

One-way function of the synapses; neuronal models.   Although it has not yet been stated explicitly, it is probably already clear that chemical synapses can transmit impulses in one direction only, namely, from the presynaptic to the postsynaptic side. It is precisely this one-way, or valve-like, function of the synapse that makes ordered activity of the CNS possible. In this respect the synapses resemble the rectifier valves and the transistors of electronic apparatus, while the axons can be compared with the other electronic components, the cables, the resistors, and the capacitors. (The validity of this comparison is limited by the ability of the cell membrane to propagate regenerative action potentials.) Artificial "neurons" made up of electronic components and combinative in "neuronal circuits" are commercially available and are used to simulate neuronal networks.

Electrical synapses.   Electrical synapses in which presynaptic and postsynaptic membranes are not separated by a synaptic cleft but instead are joined together in an electrically conducting manner have been observed occasionally in the nervous systems of invertebrates and lower vertebrates (fish) but so far not in mammals. Therefore their properties will not be discussed here. The possibility that electrical synapses occur in mammalian nervous systems as well cannot be excluded, however. There is at least some evidence, gained from electron microscope studies, to support this possibility. Neuronal contact points have been described in various parts of the brain as having the morphological criteria indicative of an electrical synapse.

Now check what you have learned.

Q 3.8   At approximately what membrane potential is the equilibrium
         potential of the EPSP situated?
         a. At −80 mV.
         b. At −15 mV.
         c. At +40 mV.
         d. The EPSP has no equilibrium potential.

Q 3.9   What area of the nerve cell surface has the lowest threshold for
         a propagated action potential?
         a. The dendrites.
         b. The soma.
         c. The axon hillock.
         d. The axon.
         e. All these areas have the same threshold.

Q 3.10   The total duration of an EPSP is approximately
         a. 2 msec.
         b. 15 msec.
         c. 100 msec.
         d. 500 msec.

Q 3.11   Which of the following events takes place at the subsynaptic
         membrane of an excitatory synapse of a motoneuron during the
         action of the excitatory transmitter substance?
         a. Increase in Na^+ permeability.
         b. Decrease in K^+ permeability.
         c. The permeability to cations remains unchanged.
         d. Large anions pass through the membrane.
         e. Local hyperpolarization.

3.4   Central Inhibitory Synapses

The importance of inhibitory processes for the normal functioning
of the CNS can be illustrated clearly by the following experiment: if
several milligrams of strychnine (a drug that blocks inhibitory synapses but leaves excitatory synapses quite unaffected) is injected into an
animal, within a few minutes severe convulsions set in, which finally
lead to death. It is scarcely possible to demonstrate in a more impres-
sive way that inhibition is a fundamental process of central nervous
activity and is just as important as excitation.

We know of two types of inhibition. In the case of *postsynaptic
inhibition* the excitability of the soma and the dendrites of the
neurons is reduced, while in the case of *presynaptic inhibition* the
release of transmitter substance at the presynaptic terminals is either
reduced or abolished. Postsynaptic inhibition seems to play the more

important role in the CNS of vertebrates. Presynaptic inhibition occurs mainly in the presynaptic terminals of somatic and visceral afferents and not so much in the rest of the nervous system.

Inhibitory postsynaptic potentials in the motoneuron. It has long been known from measurements of reflex contractions that stimulation of muscle spindle afferents not only excites the homonymous motoneurons (Fig. 3-10) but also, at the same time, inhibits the motoneurons of the antagonistic muscle. For example, stimulation of the muscle spindle afferents of the M. biceps, which flexes the elbow, simultaneously inhibits the antagonist, the M. triceps, which extends the elbow. Details of this reflex pathway will be given in the next chapter.

Figure 3-11 was recorded with an experimental arrangement similar to that illustrated on the left in Fig. 3-10 and shows the changes in membrane potential recorded with a microelectrode in a motoneuron when antagonistic muscle spindle afferents are stimulated. The resting potential of the motoneuron is -70 mV. At arrows A–D the antagonistic muscle nerve is stimulated with increasing intensity. Every stimulus triggers a *hyperpolarizing* potential change, and with the selected stimulus strengths, the maximum amplitudes of the hyperpolarizations increase in steps of 1 mV. It can be seen that the time course of the potential change is independent of the amplitude of potential change and is very similar to the time course of the EPSP. Due to the hyperpolarization, the membrane potential is shifted away from the threshold for initiating propagated action potentials, that is, the motoneuron is *inhibited*. The hyperpolarizations recorded in Fig. 3-11 are therefore termed *inhibitory postsynaptic potentials*, or *IPSP*s for short.

Ionic mechanism of the IPSP. The time course of an IPSP is practically a mirror image of that of an EPSP, with a rise time of 1 to 2 msec, a decline of about 10 msec, and a total duration therefore of

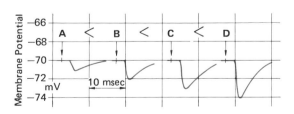

Fig. 3-11. Inhibitory postsynaptic potentials. Experimental arrangement as in Fig. 3-10, except that here an antagonistic nerve is stimulated.

approximately 12 msec. It can already be concluded from this that here, as at the end plate and the excitatory synapse, the subsynaptic change in membrane permeability that leads to the appearance of the IPSPs is short and lasts about 1 to 2 msec. This assumption has been confirmed by further experiments and mathematical analysis of the time course.

The most important experimental method of determining the ionic mechanism of the IPSP is to measure its equilibrium potential, that is, the membrane potential at which activation of the inhibitory synapses fails to evoke a potential change. The experimental setup is shown in the left half of Fig. 3-12 and is similar to that in Fig. 3-6. In this case, however, the two single microelectrodes are replaced by a double-barreled microelectrode, for it would otherwise be practically impossible to insert both electrodes into the same motoneuron located several millimeters beneath the surface of the spinal cord.

It can be seen that an IPSP triggered at a membrane potential of −65 mV (the resting potential of this cell) has an amplitude of 5 mV in a hyperpolarizing direction. If the membrane potential is lowered by a current applied through a microelectrode, the amplitude of the IPSP (at the same peripheral stimulus) increases greatly. This means that the driving force for the IPSP becomes greater during depolarization of the membrane potential. Conversely, when the membrane potential is increased, the amplitudes of the IPSPs initially become smaller and finally drop to zero at approximately −80 mV. At still higher membrane potentials the direction of the IPSP is reversed. The

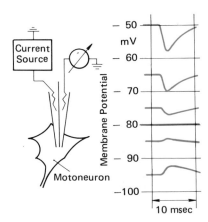

Fig. 3-12. Equilibrium potential of the IPSP. Experimental setup as in Fig. 3-11. The membrane potential of the motoneuron can be varied by applying current through the second barrel of the double-barreled microelectrode.

equilibrium potential of the IPSP, E_{IPSP}, is thus situated at -80 mV. Since the equilibrium potential for K^+ (E_K) is at about -90 mV and since that for Cl^- (E_{Cl}) is at the resting potential, the equilibrium potential of the IPSP, E_{IPSP}, is situated approximately halfway between the two.

The value of the equilibrium potential of the IPSP thus indicates that during the action of the inhibitory transmitter on the subsynaptic membrane, there is a *large increase in the permeability to K^+ and Cl^- ions*. Further experiments confirmed this conclusion. One such experiment involved electrophoretic injection into the cells of large numbers of anions and cations through multibarreled microelectrodes followed by measurements of the resulting changes in the IPSP. It was found that small cations as well as small anions can pass through the activated subsynaptic membrane of inhibitory synapses, while ions whose diameter is larger than that of the hydrated K^+ ions (for example, Na^+ ions) cannot. From these and similar test results at other synapses, the general theory has been developed that the transmitters open *pores* of a certain width at the subsynaptic membranes. All ions with a diameter smaller than that of the pores can pass through. If, in addition, the wall of the pore is electrically charged, this charge acts as a diffusion barrier for ions of the same polarity. Thus a negatively charged pore would only let through cations, but no anions, and a positively charged pore would only let anions through. It remains to be seen how far these theories are borne out in fact.

Inhibitory transmitters and their release. Just as we do not know the transmitter substance involved at the excitatory synapses, we are also unable to identify the transmitter substance(s) of the inhibitory synapses of the vertebrate CNS. On the other hand, there is a great deal of evidence to suggest that certain amino acids, particularly glycine, act as inhibitory transmitters. It is likely that there are several inhibitory transmitters. The fact that not all the inhibitory synapses are influenced pharmacologically in the same way lends support to this theory. So far it has been possible to identify beyond all reasonable doubt only one amino acid (γ-aminobutyric acid, GABA) as the transmitter substance at an inhibitory synapse of crustacea.

The mechanism of transmitter release at inhibitory synapses is probably very similar to that at excitatory synapses. Synaptic vesicles are present in the presynaptic terminals of inhibitory synapses, just as in the presynaptic terminals of excitatory synapses, and in all other respects the two types of synapses are morphologically identical. So far, miniature IPSPs have rarely been observed, which is probably because the resting potential and the E_{IPSP} are very close together: a single quantum of inhibitory transmitter substance causes only a very small change in potential which cannot be measured by the recording system.

Two poisons are known to block synaptic transmission at inhibitory synapses and thereby cause convulsions. These are strychnine, which competitively displaces the inhibitory transmitter substance at the subsynaptic membrane (cf. effect of curare at the end plate), and tetanus toxin, which probably prevents the release of the transmitter substance from the inhibitory presynaptic terminals (cf. Mg$^+$ effect and botulinus toxin effect at the end plate). Since a manifest tetanus infection usually results in death, an active preventive vaccination is generally recommended.

Inhibitory effects of the IPSP. As stated above, the hyperpolarization occurring during the IPSP shifts the membrane potential away from the threshold for a propagated action potential and thus inhibits the neuron. The inhibitory effects of the IPSP will now be examined in more detail, and particular attention will be paid to the question of whether the hyperpolarization is solely responsible for the inhibition. If this were so, then an IPSP triggered at E_{IPSP}, that is, at −80 mV, would have no inhibitory effect at all on the neuron!

Typical IPSPs and EPSPs can be seen in Fig. 3-13A. The maximum amplitudes are 2 and 3 mV, respectively. Figure 3-13B shows how the

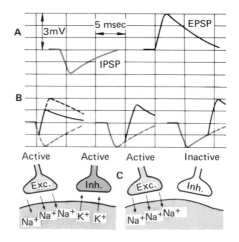

Fig. 3-13. Effect of IPSP on EPSP. Experimental arrangement as in Figs. 3-10 and 3-11. Stimulation of the antagonistic nerve gives the IPSP at A. Stimulation of the homonymous nerve gives the EPSP. In B the EPSP was triggered about 1, 3, and 5 msec after the start of the IPSP. C is a sketch of the subsynaptic changes in permeability that occur when excitatory and inhibitory synapses are activated simultaneously (left) and when only the excitatory synapse is activated.

amplitude of the EPSP behaves when it is triggered at different times during the IPSP. If, in B, the EPSP is evoked 5 or 3 msec after the start of the IPSP (center and right-hand recordings in B), then its maximum amplitude is exactly as large as that of the control EPSP in A. The inhibitory effect of the IPSP is dependent in this case solely on the shift in the membrane potential in a hyperpolarizing direction, that is, away from the threshold for a propagated action potential. If, however, in B (left-hand recording) the EPSP is evoked in the first millisecond after the start of the IPSP, the resulting EPSP is smaller than the control EPSP. Thus simple addition, such as can be observed at later points in time, does not occur. That is, during the action of the inhibitory transmitter substance on the subsynaptic membrane the inhibitory effect of the IPSP is greater than during the passive electrotonic decline of the IPSP to the resting potential.

The sketches in Fig. 3-13C show the reason for the different effectiveness of the IPSP during and after the active phase. In the left-hand sketch, the excitatory and the inhibitory synapses are activated at approximately the same time, and the inflow of Na^+ ions at the subsynaptic membrane of the excitatory synapse is partially compensated for by the simultaneous outflow of K^+ ions at the inhibitory synapse. The resulting change in potential in a depolarizing direction is therefore smaller than at the moment shown at the right in Fig. 3-13C, where the inhibitory synapse is inactive. The increase in permeability beneath the activated inhibitory subsynaptic membrane, therefore, can also be regarded as an increase in the conductance or, conversely, as a decrease in the resistance of the membrane. For a given shift in charge (for example, the Na^+ ions in Fig. 3-13C) this increase in conductance leads to a smaller potential change at the membrane. The membrane is "short-circuited" by the increase in permeability.

According to the description given so far, the Cl^- ions play only a small role in the generation of the IPSP. This is correct so long as the IPSP is initiated at the normal resting potential because E_{Cl} is situated at the resting potential. However, if the IPSP starts from a depolarized membrane potential (for example, during an EPSP), the increased Cl^- permeability will give rise to an increased inflow of Cl^- ions, contributing to the larger IPSPs which can be seen, for example, in Fig. 3-12.

If the membrane potential is situated at E_{IPSP}, activation of inhibitory synapses does not lead to a potential change. However, during the increase in subsynaptic permeability the cell is inhibited by the increased conductance of the membrane. During this time each shift in charge is at least partially compensated by the opposite shift in charge, which set in below the inhibitory subsynaptic membrane (see

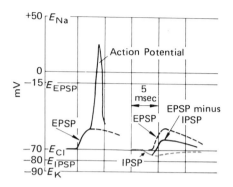

Fig. 3-14. Effect of IPSP on action potential. Experimental arrangement as in Fig. 3-13. The homonymous nerve is stimulated to such an extent that a suprathreshold EPSP is generated (on the left). On the right, the antagonistic nerve is stimulated about 3 msec before the homonymous nerve. The equilibrium potentials of Na^+, K^+, Cl^-, EPSP, and IPSP are shown.

Fig. 3-13C). When a large number of inhibitory synapses are repetitively and asynchronously activated, the postsynaptic membrane can be practically short-circuited by the large increases in conductance that occur, so that even large excitatory currents produce only small depolarizations.

The excitatory and the inhibitory synaptic events occurring at the membrane of central neurons are summarized in Fig. 3-14. The E_{EPSP} is situated at approximately -15 mV. Activation of the excitatory subsynaptic membrane thus leads to a depolarization that may perhaps reach the threshold (EPSP on left) and then evoke a propagated action potential at the axon hillock. The equilibrium potential of the IPSP is about -80 mV. The permeability for K^+ and Cl^- ions is increased beneath the activated inhibitory subsynaptic membrane, and this results in a hyperpolarization (red curve on right). Because of the IPSP, the EPSP no longer reaches the threshold, and the cell is inhibited.

Presynaptic inhibition. In the case of presynaptic inhibition, there is no change in the postsynaptic membrane, but instead the inhibitory process brings about a reduction in the release of transmitter substance at the presynaptic terminal of the excitatory synapse, i.e. an event similar to that with which we are familiar at the end plate when Mg^{++} is added or when poisoning by botulinus toxin has occurred. Presynaptic inhibition is evoked by activation of axo-axonic synapses.

In Fig. 3-15 axon 1 forms an axo-somatic synapse with neuron 3, while axon 2 forms an axo-axonal synapse with axon 1. According to

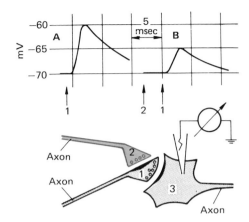

Fig. 3-15. Presynaptic inhibition of a motoneuron. Experimental setup as in Fig. 3-10. See text for further explanation.

the arrangement of the synaptic vesicles and the thick portions of the subsynaptic membrane, axon 1 is presynaptic to neuron 3 and axon 2 is presynaptic to axon 1. Activation of the synaptic ending 1 (arrow in Fig. 3-15A) evokes an EPSP of approximately 10 mV in neuron 3. The axo-somatic synapse is thus an excitatory synapse. If axon 2 is activated before axon 1 (arrows in Fig. 3-15B), the amplitude of the EPSP is only 5 mV, although no IPSP occurs at the postsynaptic membrane of cell 3. This form of EPSP inhibition *without* any change in the properties of the postsynaptic membrane is called *presynaptic inhibition*. The time course of this inhibition is about 100 to 150 msec and is thus much longer than that of the IPSP.

It is not known what subsynaptic changes in permeability are triggered by activation of the axo-axonal synapse, nor is it known what transmitter substance is released at axon 2. All that is certain is that activation of the axo-axonal synapse reduces the amount of transmitter substance released at the axo-somatic synapse. The current hypothesis is that this is probably brought about by a reduction in the amplitude of the presynaptic action potential in ending 1. Depolarization of axon 1 can in fact be observed during presynaptic inhibition. Since depolarization of the membrane potential leads to a reduced action potential amplitude, and since the release of transmitter substance is partly dependent on this amplitude, an action potential invading ending 1 during presynaptic inhibition will release less transmitter substance and thus evoke a small EPSP. In an extreme case (for example, repeated activation), ending 1 may become so depolarized following activation of the axo-axonal synapse that it is no longer possible for an action potential to be propagated; therefore only a very reduced electrotonically conducted action potential reaches the ending, resulting in only very little if any transmitter release.

In the CNS of mammals presynaptic inhibition occurs chiefly at the excitatory synapses that are formed by the endings of afferent fibers in the spinal cord. If, for example, neuron 3 in Fig. 3-15 is a motoneuron, then axon 1 is an afferent fiber from a muscle spindle, while axon 2 originates from a central interneuron. Functionally speaking, presynaptic inhibition of primary afferent fibers provides a possibility to control the sensory inflow from the periphery at the earliest possible site in the CNS. This aspect of presynaptic inhibition will be described in more detail in Chapter 7.

Check your knowledge by answering the following questions:

Q 3.12 At approximately what membrane potential is the equilibrium potential of the IPSP situated?
    a. At -90 mV.
    b. At -70 mV.
    c. At -15 mV.
    d. At $+40$ mV.
    e. None of these values is correct.

Q 3.13 The total duration of an IPSP is
    a. 1–2 msec.
    b. 10–12 msec.
    c. 100 msec.
    d. 200 msec.

Q 3.14 An IPSP inhibits a neuron because
    a. it hyperpolarizes the membrane potential.
    b. it leads to a reduction in the amount of transmitter substance released at excitatory synapses.
    c. it changes the threshold of the neuron.
    d. it increases the conductance of the membrane.
    e. All these events occur during an IPSP.

Q 3.15 Depolarization of a nerve cell to -50 mV
    a. considerably shortens the duration of the EPSP.
    b. increases the amplitude of the IPSP.
    c. impedes generation of an EPSP.
    d. increases the amplitude of the EPSP.
    e. leaves EPSP and IPSP unchanged.
    f. None of the preceding statements is correct.

4

THE PHYSIOLOGY OF SMALL GROUPS
OF NEURONS; REFLEXES

Axonal impulse conduction and excitatory and inhibitory synaptic transmission are the two fundamental processes of neuronal activity. The complex abilities of the brain are achieved primarily by suitable connections between groups of neurons. In the first part of this chapter we shall examine some typical neuronal networks of a type constantly recurring in various sections of the brain. Some of these networks are used to boost weak signals; others serve to suppress overactivity (Sec. 4.1). These networks resemble the integrated circuits in electronics, that is, prefabricated circuits that can be used in a wide variety of electronic equipment. Their tasks include the suppression and the boosting of signals. In electronic apparatus, and also in the central nervous system, components of this type are used to maintain, as far as possible, optimum operating conditions.

Then we shall study simple (Sec. 4.2) and more complex reflex arcs (Sec. 4.3). By reflex arcs we mean complete neuronal networks extending from the peripheral receptor through the CNS to the peripheral effector. They serve to perform reliably and with a minimum of effort the constantly recurring stereotyped reactions of the organism to its environment.

4.1 Typical Neuronal Circuits

In this section we shall proceed from the long-established fact that sooner or later after their emergence from the soma, the axons of most neurons subdivide into a few or many collateral branches that form synapses with several to many other neurons. This process is referred to as *divergence*. Correspondingly, most neurons receive synapses from a large number of neurons. This phenomenon has been termed *convergence*. Because of the extensive divergence and convergence in the CNS it is quite correct to say that each neuron is connected with every other neuron, even though the connection may be mediated through many interneurons. One should, however, be aware that these connections are not arbitrary and chaotic but follow definite circuit plans that surpass in finesse and efficiency those of large, modern pieces of electronic equipment.

Temporal and *spatial facilitation* are the two simplest methods of turning subthreshold excitations into suprathreshold ones, that is, of boosting neuronal activity. We shall therefore discuss these mechanisms after we have examined the phenomena of divergence and convergence. Then we shall turn our attention to three typical *inhibitory circuits* that improve the efficiency of the CNS by suppressing undesired activity. Finally, to complete the picture, we shall learn about two possible ways of maintaining activity, or at least simplifying its repetition, once it has been induced in the CNS; that is, we shall be looking at events that may play a role in learning or remembering.

Divergence and convergence. The afferent fibers of peripheral receptors enter the spinal cord via the dorsal root and then divide into a large number of collaterals that lead to spinal neurons. A diagram of this process of *divergence* is given in Fig. 4-1. Divergence serves to make afferent information accessible simultaneously to various sections of the CNS, for example, to the motoneurons, the cerebellum, or the cerebral cortex. An action potential coming from a single receptor afferent can be considerably strengthened as a result of the subdivision of the axon into a large number of collaterals, that is, as a result of divergence. This division of the dorsal root fibers into a large number of collaterals is only one example of divergence, which occurs in nearly all parts of the CNS.

It is extremely difficult to assess divergence quantitatively because it is almost always impossible, either with histological or physiological methods, to trace all the collaterals of a neuron. However, the motoaxons are exceptions worth mentioning here. They emerge from the spinal cord in the ventral roots and lead to the muscles where they divide into collaterals that innervate a varying number of muscle fibers. Since each muscle fiber is innervated by only one collateral, the average divergence of each motoaxon can be calculated from the number of motoaxons and muscle fibers present in a muscle. In humans values between 1:15 (external eye muscles) and 1:1900 (muscles of extremities) and more are found. (In addition, the motoaxons give off collaterals while they are still in the spinal cord, that is, before they enter the ventral roots, but we do not know exactly how many.)

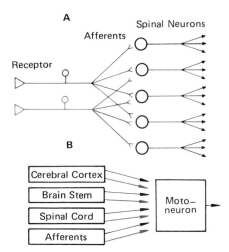

Fig. 4-1. A: Diagram of the divergence of two dorsal root fibers (afferents) to spinal neurons. The axons of these neurons in turn branch into a large number of collaterals. B: Diagram of excitatory (black arrows) and inhibitory (red arrows) afferents converging onto a motoneuron. The motoneuron forms the final common pathway of all motor reflexes.

Figure 4-1A shows two afferent fibers whose axons diverge in each case to four neurons. As a result, three of the total five neurons shown are connected to both afferent fibers or, seen the other way round, two afferent fibers *converge* on each neuron. Many dozens to several thousands of axons converge on most neurons in the CNS. Let us take the example of the motoneuron to make this clear. On the average, about 6,000 axon collaterals terminate on the motoneuron. As summarized in Fig. 4-1B these axon collaterals come not only from the periphery but also from neurons of the spinal cord, the brain stem, and the cerebral cortex. Some form excitatory (black arrows) and others inhibitory (red arrows) synapses.

Since several thousand axon collaterals converge on the motoneurons, it is easy to see that whether or not a motoneuron discharges a propagated action potential depends on the sum and the direction of the synaptic processes effective at any one time. In this sense the motoneuron (and many other neurons) processes, or integrates, the excitatory and inhibitory events occurring at its membrane. Long before the discovery of EPSPs and IPSPs the integrative function of the motoneurons was known from studies of muscle contractions after peripheral and central electric stimulation. Around the turn of the century the English physiologist Sherrington had already described the motoneuron as the "final common pathway" of the motor system, that is, as the cell that weighs all the excitatory and the inhibitory influences, one against the other. Action potentials are discharged only when the excitatory influences predominate, or in modern terms, for as long as suprathreshold EPSPs occur.

   Temporal and spatial facilitation, occlusion.   On the left in Fig. 4-2A is shown an experimental arrangement for testing the effect exerted on a neuron by repetitive stimulation of an axon. A single stimulus (arrow, top right) induces a typical EPSP with a total duration of approximately 15 msec. When two stimuli are applied at an interval of approximately 4 msec (arrows, center right) the second EPSP begins before the first has fully decayed. As a result, the cell is more strongly depolarized, and the membrane potential approaches more closely the threshold. A third EPSP occurring 4 msec later (arrows, bottom right in Fig. 4-2A) reaches threshold, and a propagated action potential occurs. EPSPs triggered rapidly one after the other have an additive excitatory effect on a neuron. This type of increase in excitability brought about by successive EPSPs is therefore termed *temporal facilitation*. Temporal facilitation through an axon is only possible because the duration of the EPSP is longer than the refractory period of the axons. Temporal facilitation is of great

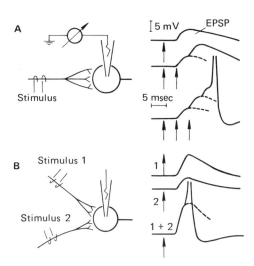

Fig. 4-2.   Facilitation in the nervous system. *A*: Temporal facilitation. A single stimulus (one arrow) and paired stimuli (two arrows, time between stimuli about 4 msec) generate subthreshold EPSPs; the third stimulus (three arrows) evokes an action potential. *B*: Spatial facilitation. Stimulus 1 and stimulus 2 each trigger a subthreshold EPSP. Simultaneous stimulation of both axons evokes an action potential.

physiological importance because many nervous processes, for example, receptor discharges, occur repetitively and as a result can summate to produce suprathreshold depolarizations at synapses.

The experimental setup in Fig. 4-2B demonstrates the occurrence of *spatial facilitation*: stimulus 1 alone generates a subthreshold EPSP (top right in B) and stimulus 2 alone (center right) also gives a subthreshold EPSP. But if 1 and 2 are stimulated simultaneously (bottom right), the threshold is reached, and a propagated action potential is elicited. Joint stimulation of 1 and 2 thus leads to a propagated action potential, that is, to a process that could not be evoked by the individual EPSPs alone. Expressed generally, *facilitation*, whether temporal or spatial, exists when more propagated action potentials occur than correspond to the sum of the individual effects.

This general definition of facilitation is illustrated in Fig. 4-3A–C. The circles symbolize neurons. Filled circles denote a suprathreshold EPSP; half-filled circles indicate a subthreshold EPSP. As in Fig. 4-1A, two afferent receptor populations should make partially overlapping contact (convergence) with the 12 neurons in each of A to C. Diagram A shows what happens when one receptor population is

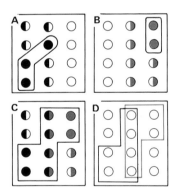

Fig. 4-3. *A–C*: Spatial facilitation. The population, consisting of twelve neurons, possesses four neurons that may be excited by two different afferent inputs (center row of neurons in A to C). Input A evokes subthreshold EPSPs in three of these four neurons (A, half-filled circles) and an action potential in one neuron (filled circle). Input B induces subthreshold EPSPs in these four neurons. Simultaneous activity (C) of inputs A and B leads to suprathreshold excitation of all neurons common to A and B. Thus the number of neurons excited to above the threshold is larger than the sum of the neurons excited by the single stimuli 8 > 3 + 2. D. Occlusion. If each input produces a suprathreshold excitation of all four neurons common to both inputs (black and red framed neurons in D), the simultaneous activation of both inputs results in a number of activated neurons that is smaller than the sum of the neurons excited by each input alone, 8 < 6 + 6.

stimulated; we get subthreshold EPSPs in five neurons and suprathreshold EPSPs in three neurons. Stimulation of the other receptor
population, as *B* shows, leads to a propagated action potential in two
neurons and to subthreshold EPSPs in six neurons. Of the latter, four
neurons are identical with the neurons excited by receptor population
A. If both receptor populations are stimulated simultaneously, then a
suprathreshold excitation is triggered in not only 3 + 2 = 5 but a total
of eight neurons (*C*). Thus, more neurons undergo suprathreshold
excitation than the total number of neurons with suprathreshold excitation in the case of the two single stimuli. As already stated we call
this process *facilitation*, and in this case it is spatial facilitation.

It can also happen, however, that when stimulated separately, both
receptor populations excite the center row of neurons beyond the
threshold. This situation is indicated by the black and the red framing
in Fig. 4-3*D*. Each individual stimulus thus excites six neurons above
the threshold. If, under these conditions, both receptor populations in
Fig. 4-3*D* are stimulated simultaneously, then not 6 + 6 = 12 neurons
but only eight neurons are excited above the threshold. This phenomenon is referred to as *occlusion*. The process of facilitation illustrated
in *A–C* has thus turned into occlusion as a result of an increase in the
excitability of the neurons involved (for example, if additional excitatory effects act on the neurons).

Let us recapitulate: if the success of several simultaneous stimuli
or of several stimuli occurring in rapid succession is greater than the
sum of the individual stimuli, then we term this *facilitation*. If the
success of the stimuli is less than the sum of the individual stimuli,
then we call this *occlusion*.

Simple inhibitory circuits. Pharmacological elimination of the
inhibitory processes of the CNS (strychnine, tetanus toxin) leads to
convulsions and death. Quite clearly, inhibitory circuits serve to suppress superfluous and excessive excitatory effects. This task is taken
care of mainly by circuits that act back on the excitation itself: as the
original excitation becomes stronger it is inhibited more strongly. In
electronics such circuits are known as "negative feedback circuits." In
addition, there are inhibitory circuits that, during an excitatory event,
automatically suppress any opposing excitatory events or ensure that
an excitation remains unaffected by any neighboring activity. We will
now examine these various inhibitory circuits that are characteristic of
the CNS.

As mentioned previously the afferents of the stretch receptors of
muscle spindles (called Ia fibers) form excitatory synapses at their
homonymous motoneurons and inhibitory synapses with antagonistic

motoneurons. In the latter case an interneuron is interposed between
the Ia fiber and the motoneuron. This situation is represented in Fig.
4-4*A*. The inhibition is termed *antagonistic inhibition*. Here (and in *B*
and *C*) the inhibitory interneurons are shown in red. If, for example,
the Ia afferents from the muscle spindles of a flexor muscle are activated (arrows in Fig. 4-4*A*), they then excite the motoneurons of the
homonymous flexor muscle and inhibit the motoneurons of the extensor muscles acting on the same joint. In physiological terms, this
antagonistic inhibition is extremely useful because it automatically,
that is, without any additional voluntary or involuntary control, assists
the movement of the joints.

   In Figure 4-4*A* the antagonistic inhibition suppresses excitatory
events without influencing the excitatory process by which it was
generated. Therefore there is no feedback to the source of the excitation. On the other hand, the inhibitory interneurons in Fig. 4-4*B* act
back on the cells by which they themselves were activated. In this
case there is negative feedback, and this inhibition is termed *feedback
inhibition*. The motoneurons provide a particularly clear example of
such a feedback inhibition. As Fig. 4-4*B* shows, the motoaxons give off
collaterals to inhibitory interneurons whose axons in turn form inhibitory synapses on motoneurons. This inhibition is called *Renshaw
inhibition* after its discoverer, and the inhibitory interneurons are
called *Renshaw cells*. As the motoneurons become more excited, the
Renshaw cells also become more excited, resulting in greater inhibition of the motoneurons after a short latent period (one interneuron).
This guarantees that weak motoneuron activity is transmitted undisturbed to the muscles while excessive activity is damped to prevent
hyperactivity of the muscles or even convulsions.

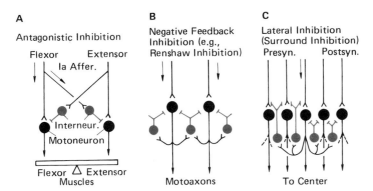

Fig. 4-4. Typical inhibitory circuits. The inhibitory interneurons are
shown in red in all three neuronal circuits. See text for detailed description.

A similar form of inhibitory feedback circuit frequently encountered in the CNS is illustrated in Fig. 4-4C. The inhibitory interneurons are connected in such a way that they act not only back on the excited cell itself (arrow) but also on neighboring cells with the same function and in such a manner that these cells are particularly strongly inhibited. This type of inhibition is called *lateral inhibition* because it ensures that an inhibited zone is generated lateral to the excited zone. Excitation is thus surrounded on all sides by an inhibited field; therefore this phenomenon is also referred to as *surround inhibition.* Surround inhibition, or lateral inhibition, plays a particularly important role in afferent systems where it may be mediated by both postsynaptic (Fig. 4-4C, right) and presynaptic (Fig. 4-4C, left) inhibitory synapses. Its advantages are described in detail in Chapter 7.

Positive feedback and posttetanic potentiation.   The great importance of inhibitory circuits for the normal functioning of the CNS has been demonstrated experimentally on many occasions, and they are a generally accepted feature. On the other hand, the view is often advanced (also, the object of much dissent) that the CNS also contains positive feedback circuits, which, by feeding back excitation to already excited cells, would cause the excitation to move in a circle (reverberating excitation). An excitatory feedback circuit of this type is illustrated in Fig. 4-5A. It could serve to maintain an induced activity for a long time. Many people say that short-term memory is due to the reverberating of excitation in such positive feedback circuits, yet there is almost no experimental evidence to support this. For the present, therefore, the question must remain unanswered as to whether or not positive feedback circuits exist in the CNS, and if they do, what physiological importance they might have.

There is another, better known way of facilitating the repetition of neuronal activity. Repeated (repetitive, tetanic) use of a synapse often results in a considerable increase in the synaptic potentials, a phenomenon referred to as *posttetanic potentiation.* For example, in the experiment illustrated in Fig. 4-5B, single stimuli gave EPSPs of approximately 4 mV amplitude (control values at left). After brief tetanic stimulation (duration 1 min, frequency 100/sec = 6,000 stimuli) the amplitude of the EPSP was approximately 11 mV, that is, about 275 percent of the initial value. This posttetanic potentiation at first usually declines at a fast rate, then more slowly, and, finally, in the example shown, it disappears after about 3.5 to 4 min. The duration and the extent of posttetanic potentiation depend very much on the synapse under investigation and on the duration and the frequency of the repetitive stimulation. The longest known posttetanic

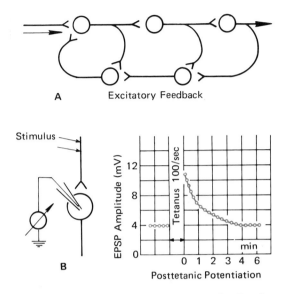

Fig. 4-5. *A*: Neuronal circuit giving positive feedback. When suitably dimensioned this hypothetical circuit could lead to reverberating of excitation. *B*: Posttetanic potentiation. Experimental arrangement illustrated at left. Presynaptic axon stimulated by regularly repeated single stimuli. In between, the axon is stimulated for 1 min at a frequency of 100/sec (= 6,000 stimuli). The time shown on the abscissa in the right-hand graph indicates the time after the end of the tetanus.

potentiations last several hours. It is perhaps significant that particularly long posttetanic potentiations are found in the hippocampus, a central nervous structure that is assumed to play a special role in memory and learning.

What changes at the synapse are responsible for the improved transmission following repetitive activation? Practically any of the links in the long chain of processes occurring during activation of a chemical synapse (see Chapter 3) could be responsible, but it has been proved experimentally that there are essentially two main *presynaptic mechanisms* to which this improvement may be ascribed.

First, repetitive activation of the presynaptic axon membrane leads to an increase (hyperpolarization) of the resting potential and thus to an increase in the *amplitude of the action potential*. The increased action potential releases more transmitter substance into the synaptic cleft. This process is approximately the reverse of what happens during presynaptic inhibition, where, as we have seen, a reduction in the amplitude of the presynaptic action potential leads to less transmitter substance being released.

Second, repetitive activation gives rise to increased availability of transmitter at the synaptic gap. This *mobilization* of transmitter substance also causes improved synaptic transmission because a greater portion of the transmitter substance stored in the presynaptic terminal is released per action potential.

Q 4.1 Turn again to Fig. 4-2A. How does a reduction in the stimulus frequency affect the temporal facilitation?
   a. It improves it.
   b. It makes it weaker.
   c. It has no effect.

Q 4.2 In a neuronal population, activation of one nerve leads to suprathreshold excitation of 22 neurons, while activation of another nerve results in suprathreshold excitation of 10 neurons. Combined simultaneous activation of both neurons causes suprathreshold activation of 32 neurons. Would you call this process facilitation or occlusion?

Q 4.3 Which of the following factors seem chiefly responsible for post-tetanic potentiation?
   a. Increased synthesis of transmitter.
   b. Increased availability of transmitter at the synaptic cleft.
   c. Slower breakdown of transmitter in the synaptic cleft.
   d. Increased sensitivity of the postsynaptic membrane.
   e. Increased postsynaptic action potentials.

Q 4.4 Lateral inhibition (surround inhibition)
   a. cannot be regarded as a feedback circuit.
   b. is an example of positive feedback in the CNS.
   c. acts like negative feedback.
   d. causes particularly weak inhibition in neighboring cells of the same function.
   e. is mediated exclusively by presynaptic synapses.

4.2   The Monosynaptic Reflex Arc

Receptors are the sensors that permit the organism to detect changes in its environment or within itself and thus to provide a basis for appropriate action. In many cases the afferent fibers of the receptors are connected in such a way in the CNS that their activation always leads to certain stereotyped reactions of the organism. In the course of phylogenic or individual development, these reactions have proved to be particularly appropriate responses. Such stereotyped reactions of the CNS to sensory stimuli are called *reflexes*. You will undoubtedly be able to supply a large number of examples yourselves. Touching a hot object makes us withdraw our hand, even before we are aware of any pain and can take any conscious action. Touching the cornea of the eye always triggers a blink (corneal reflex). Foreign bodies in the windpipe make us cough. When food comes into contact with the posterior pharyngeal wall, a swallowing reflex is triggered, and so on.

Most reflexes occur without our being consciously aware of them: for example, the reflexes that are responsible for the passage or processing of food in the stomach and intestinal tract, or those that continuously adapt circulation and respiration to the required levels. Nor are we normally aware of any of the motor reflexes that day in and day out maintain the upright posture of our bodies in space, keep our balance, and, through appropriate regulatory reactions, permit us to carry out voluntary movements successfully. Of the large number of reflex arcs involved in controlling the motor system, we will examine only the simplest, namely, the monosynaptic reflex arc of the stretch reflex, which, despite its simple structural plan, is probably the most important motor reflex. We will start by discussing the receptor organ of this reflex arc, the muscle spindle.

The muscle spindle. Each muscle contains a number of muscle fibers which are thinner and shorter than the ordinary muscle fibers. Usually, several of these fibers are grouped together and, as shown in Fig. 4-6, are encased in a connective tissue capsule. Because of its shape this structure is called a *muscle spindle*. The muscle fibers inside the capsule are called *intrafusal* muscle fibers, while the ordinary muscle fibers, which constitute the major part of the muscle, are called *extrafusal* fibers. To give some idea of the dimensions we might note at this point that the intrafusal fibers are between approximately 15 and 30 μ in diameter and 4 to 7 mm long. The extrafusal

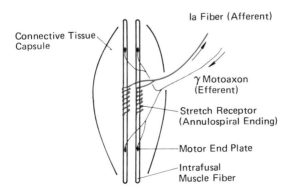

Fig. 4-6. Highly simplified schematic diagram of a muscle spindle. See text for detailed description.

muscle fibers are about 50 to 100 μ in diameter and vary in length from several millimeters to many centimeters and even tens of centimeters (more details are given in Chapter 5).

The intrafusal muscle fibers, just as the extrafusal fibers, possess a motor innervation. The motoaxons of intrafusal muscle fibers are also thinner than normal motoaxons. The latter are usually called Aα fibers, abbreviated to α *fibers* (α = alpha), while the motoaxons of the intrafusal musculature are called Aγ fibers, abbreviated to γ *fibers* (γ = gamma). (α fibers are 12 to 21 μ in diameter and γ fibers 2 to 8 μ. It is not known whether the relationship thick muscle fiber = thick axon, thin muscle fiber = thin axon is coincidental or causal.) The γ motoaxons form synaptic connections, similar to end plates, on the intrafusal muscle fibers, which, as Fig. 4-6 shows, are usually located in each lateral third of the muscle fibers. Morphologically it is possible to distinguish between two types of intrafusal fibers, two types of γ motoaxons and two types of intrafusal end-plate formations. The physiological importance of these differences is still the subject of debate, and therefore we will not go into this matter any further.

In addition to motor innervation via γ fibers, the muscle spindles also possess a sensory innervation (Fig. 4-6). These afferent fibers wind themselves several times around the center of the intrafusal muscle fibers, and this formation is thus called an *annulospiral ending*. The afferent fibers are thick, myelinated fibers (10 to 20 μ in diameter) termed *Group Ia fibers*. In each spindle the annulospiral endings are innervated by *one* Ia fiber; because of their innervation by Ia fibers the annulospiral endings are also called *primary sensory endings*.

In terms of function, the primary sensory endings of the muscle spindles are *stretch receptors*. If the muscle and the muscle spindles it contains are stretched, then action potentials are transmitted to the CNS from the annulospiral endings. The frequency of the action potentials is proportional to the degree of stretching. As the muscle spindle is stretched, that is, as it becomes longer, the impulse frequency of the muscle spindles increases. If the muscle contracts, or, more accurately, if the extrafusal muscle fibers contract, then the muscle spindles become shorter, and the impulse frequency of the Ia fibers is reduced or may even drop to zero. The muscle spindles thus signal the length of the muscle.

Many, if not all, muscle spindles also possess a further sensory innervation that is situated in general between the annulospiral ending and the motor end plates. These sensory endings are also stretch sensitive. Their afferent fibers, however, are thinner (Group II fibers) than those of the annulospiral endings. The latter are also called primary muscle spindle endings because of the Ia innervation, and similarly the receptor structures innervated by Group II fibers are also called *secondary* muscle spindle endings. Their shape is similar to that of the primary endings, but it is usually not as uniform. The functional significance of the secondary endings is still far from fully understood, and we will not go into this in any more detail here.

The monosynaptic stretch reflex.   What effect does stretching the muscle spindles have on the homonymous extrafusal musculature? It has already been stated in the discussion of central excitatory synapses, and shown in Figure 4-4A, that the Ia fibers form excitatory synapses on homonymous motoneurons. Activation of the primary muscle spindle endings by stretching the muscle must lead to excitation of the homonymous motoneurons. A sketch of an experiment to test this prediction is given in Fig. 4-7. As the curve (bottom left) shows, brief stretching of the muscle resulting from a light tap of the hammer on the recording arm produces, after a short latent period, a contraction (twitch) of the muscle. Obviously, the brief stretching of the muscle activated primary muscle spindle endings so that a volley of action potentials entered the spinal cord via the Ia fibers and (among other things) triggered *monosynaptic* EPSPs in the homonymous motoneurons. Some of these EPSPs were suprathreshold and triggered a slight muscular contraction. This reflex is called the stretch reflex. Since it possesses only *one* central synapse, namely, that of the

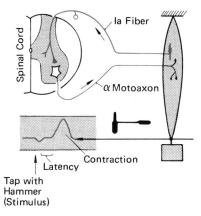

Fig. 4-7.   Reflex arc of the monosynaptic stretch reflex. A light tap with a hammer on the indicator of the measuring instrument (downward deflection in the recording trace) leads, after a short latent period, to a contraction of the muscle. The arc of this reflex is shown leading from the muscle spindles via the Ia fibers to the motoneurons and back to the muscle.

Ia fibers on the homonymous motoneurons, it is called a *monosynaptic stretch reflex*. In the case of the monosynaptic stretch reflex the receptors i.e. the muscle spindles, and the effector, namely, the extrafusal muscle fibers, are both located in the same organ—the muscle. The monosynaptic stretch reflex therefore is often referred to as the monosynaptic intrinsic reflex.

As Fig. 4-8*A* shows, a *reflex arc* consists of a peripheral receptor, an afferent fiber, one or more central neurons, an efferent fiber, and an effector. The corresponding parts of the reflex arc for the monosynaptic stretch reflex are shown in Fig. 4-8*B*. As can be seen, the monosynaptic stretch reflex (intrinsic reflex) is the simplest example of a complete reflex arc.

The best-known example of a monosynaptic stretch reflex is the *patellar reflex*: a tap on the tendon of M. quadriceps (extensor of the knee joint on the ventral side of the upper thigh) below the knee cap (patella) produces brief stretching of the M. quadriceps. After a short latent period the muscle contracts (twitches) slightly, and as a result the free-hanging lower leg is raised slightly. This test of the patellar reflex provides a check on the monosynaptic reflex arc. Failure to react or a weak or excessive reaction indicates a problem that would then have to be diagnosed by more detailed neurological examination. The fault could lie in the individual parts of the reflex arc (Fig. 4-8), but it could also be that the other inputs to the motoneurons (Fig. 4-1) are not normal and thus underexcite or overexcite the cells. Testing of the patellar and similar reflexes is a very simple way of checking motor reflex arcs.

The time between the start of the stimulus and the action of the effector is called the *reflex time*. In the case of the patellar reflex, the

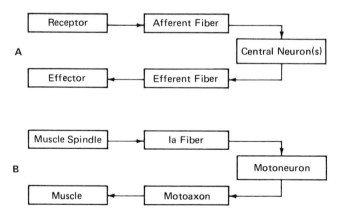

Fig. 4-8. *A*: General designations of the parts of a complete reflex arc. *B*: The parts of the arc of the monosynaptic stretch reflex.

delay between the tap with the hammer and the twitch of the muscle is scarcely noticeable to the observer, which indicates that the reflex time is very short. It is determined mainly by the conduction time of the afferent and the efferent action potentials in the Ia fibers and the α motoaxons, respectively. In an adult person the pathway from the M. quadriceps to the spinal cord and back measures approximately 80 + 80 = 160 cm. The speed of conduction in Ia fibers and α motoaxons is high, approximately 100 m/sec. The pathway of 160 cm = 1.6 m is thus traversed in 16/1,000 sec = 16 msec. In addition to this conduction time we must allow about 1 msec for each of the following: the conversion of the stretching into excitation of primary sensory endings of the muscle spindle, transmission in the synapses at the motoneurons (synaptic delay), transmission from the end plates to the muscle fibers, and triggering of contraction by the muscle fiber action potential (electromechanical coupling). Altogether the *reflex time of the monosynaptic stretch (intrinsic) reflex* is approximately 20 msec.

Role of the intrafusal muscle fibers. What is the importance of the motor innervation of the stretch receptor, that is, the muscle spindle, by the γ motoaxons? It has been seen that stretching of the extrafusal muscle fibers can also lead to stretching and thus to excitation of the primary muscle spindle endings (compare *A* with *B* in Fig. 4-9). But there is also a second way of exciting the primary muscle spindle endings: contraction of the intrafusal muscle fibers (Fig. 4-9*C*). This contraction of the intrafusal muscle fibers does not change the length and the tension of the entire muscle. It is too weak for that, even if all

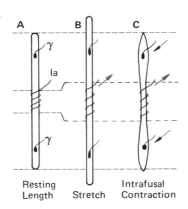

Fig. 4-9. Activation of the primary sensory (annulospiral) endings of a muscle spindle by stretching of the entire muscle (*B*) or by intrafusal contraction (*C*).

the intrafusal muscle fibers of a muscle were to contract simultaneously. However, intrafusal contraction is sufficient to stretch the central portion of the intrafusal fibers, inducing excitation in the primary sensory endings.

There are thus two ways of exciting the primary (annulospiral) endings of the muscle spindles: stretching the entire muscle and contracting the intrafusal muscle fibers. Both processes result in afferent action potentials in Group Ia fibers, generating EPSPs in the homonymous α motoneurons. Consequently, contraction of the extrafusal musculature can be triggered or at least facilitated by the muscle spindles when the muscle is stretched and the intrafusal muscle fibers contract. Both processes can also be mutually complementary or can have a mutually weakening effect: intrafusal contraction and simultaneous stretching of the whole muscle will bring about particularly strong activation of the stretch receptors.

Conversely, extrafusal contraction and simultaneous intrafusal relaxation relax the stretch receptor completely. Any desired intermediate value can be adjusted between these two extremes of maximum activity and complete inactivation by means of correspondingly graduated contractions of the intrafusal muscle fibers. In other words, the threshold of a stretch receptor can be varied by intrafusal "pretensioning." When intrafusal contraction occurs, the threshold of the stretch receptor is lowered in response to stretching of the muscle. The muscle spindle reacts more sensitively to the stretching of a muscle (further details will be given in Chapter 6).

Voluntary movements are initiated in the cerebral cortex. Accordingly, the cerebral cortex has two possible ways of triggering a contraction. On the one hand, it can excite the α motoneurons directly, and the extrafusal musculature will contract to the desired extent; on the other hand, it can first excite the γ motoneurons, which then bring about activation of the stretch reflex arc by means of intrafusal contraction, causing the extrafusal musculature to contract. This latter possibility is often termed the γ loop. It appears more complicated than the direct corticospinal activation of the α motoneurons, but it seems that precise, sensitive movements are executed by simultaneous activation of the direct α pathway and the γ loop (α-γ coactivation; see Chapter 6 for more details).

Muscle spindle and muscle tone; length control system. Our body is constantly exposed to the influence of gravity, which tends to pull us to the ground. For this reason many of our muscles, in particular the extensors of the lower limbs and also the back and the neck muscles, are kept in a certain active state of tension when we maintain an upright posture. This activity of the muscles is referred to as *tone*. For example, our knee joints would give way were it not for the fact that this tendency is counteracted by the constant tension of M. quadriceps, that is, the extensor of the knee at the anterior surface of the thigh. This continuous contraction (= tonus) of the M. quadriceps is controlled involuntarily. A decisive role in this is played by the monosynaptic stretch reflex. Every slight, undetectable bending of the knee joint leads to a stretching of the M. quadriceps and to increased activation of the stretch receptors of the muscle spindles (cf. patellar reflex). This in turn gives rise to greater activation of the α motoneurons of the M. quadriceps and to increased muscle tension which immediately counteracts the incipient bending of the joint. Conversely, too strong a contraction of the extrafusal muscle fibers leads to relaxation of the stretch receptors. Their impulse rate drops as does the flow of excitatory impulses to the motoneurons, with the result that the muscle tone weakens. In general terms, this regulatory circuit serves to maintain constant muscle *length*. The monosynaptic stretch reflex acts as a *length control system* (length servomechanism) which maintains a constant muscle length through feedback from the muscle spindles. Changes in the load on the muscle or tiredness are automatically balanced out by this mechanism. The required sensitivity of the muscle spindles, which serve as misalignment detectors in this length servomechanism, is set by contractions of intrafusal muscle fibers. If the centrally initiated activation of the γ loop is interrupted, for example, during sleep, then the stretch reflexes are reduced, and the muscle tonus decreases. A familiar example is when a person falls asleep sitting up in a chair and his head drops onto his chest (he "nods off").

Muscle spindle and movement; follow-up servomechanism. The stretch reflex can be used also to vary the length of the muscle via γ innervation of the intrafusal muscle fibers. For example, if the intrafusal muscle fibers are contracted at a certain muscle length, the primary endings are stretched and the stretch reflex is evoked. The muscle contracts until the original discharge rate of the primary spindle afferents is reached again, that is, until the muscle has contracted by about the same amount as the spindles. In this case, the stretch reflex, together with the γ loop, forms a *follow-up servomechanism* in which the muscle length follows the muscle spindle length.

The monosynaptic stretch reflex is not only involved in maintaining a given muscle length at a constant value but also plays a part in every change in muscle length. Thus, it is the most important motor reflex. The muscle spindle receptors are the sensors of a control circuit (analogy: thermometer in refrigerator), and each change in muscle length (refrigerator temperature) from the preset value (for instance, a temperature of +4 C as selected at the temperature control knob of the refrigerator) is indicated by these receptors. If the muscle stretches (temperature in refrigerator rises) then the α motoneurons are excited (the cooling unit of the refrigerator is switched on). Once the preset value is reached or exceeded, the excitation declines (cooling unit of refrigerator is switched off). Changes in the desired value via the γ loop (resetting the temperature at the control knob of the refrigerator) results in corresponding regulation of the muscle to the new desired value (refrigerator warms up or cools down). The comparison with the temperature control system does not quite stand up to critical examination because the length of a muscle is much more precisely and finely controlled than the temperature in an ordinary household refrigerator. The comparison does, however, make clear that the monosynaptic stretch reflex arc is a control circuit, which, together with the γ loop, is capable of participating very effectively in the control of our muscles.

Q 4.5 Which of the following statements about the muscle spindles are correct?
  a. The intrafusal muscle fibers are thinner and longer than the extrafusal muscle fibers.
  b. The γ motoaxons innervate the primary stretch receptors.
  c. The muscle spindles possess no innervation other than sensory innervation.
  d. Afferent volleys in the Ia fibers inhibit the homonymous motoneurons and excite their antagonists.
  e. All the above statements are correct.
  f. None of these statements is correct.

Q 4.6 Which of the following processes will bring about an increase in tonus of the extrafusal musculature via the monosynaptic stretch reflex?
  a. Passive shortening of the muscle (for example, the pendant lower part of the leg is extended by a second person, and this results in passive shortening of the M. quadriceps).
  b. Active contraction of the intrafusal muscle fibers.
  c. Stretching of the extrafusal muscle fibers.
  d. Relaxation of the intrafusal muscle fibers.
  e. Contraction of the extrafusal muscle fibers.

Q 4.7 Let us assume that the afferent and the efferent pathways of a monsynaptic stretch reflex arc are each 120 cm long (those of a foot muscle). The speed of conduction of the afferent Ia fibers is 100 m/sec and that of the α motoaxons is 80 m/sec. What is the minimum reflex time in milliseconds? Add 3 msec to the conduction times to allow for receptor activation, synaptic transmission, and neuromuscular coupling.

Q 4.8 Under what conditions are the stretch receptors of the muscle spindles more strongly excited?
  a. Contraction of the extrafusal muscle fibers with simultaneous contraction of the intrafusal muscle fibers.
  b. Contraction of the extrafusal muscle fibers with simultaneous relaxation of the intrafusal muscle fibers.

4.3   Polysynaptic Motor Reflexes

In its reflex arc, the monosynaptic stretch reflex possesses only one central neuron, the motoneuron. In all other motor reflex arcs several neurons are connected in series, and the motoneuron is always the last link in the chain of central neurons. These reflexes therefore are called *polysynaptic*. In addition, in the polysynaptic reflexes, the receptor and the effector are spatially separated in the body, so these reflexes may also be called *extrinsic reflexes.*

Polysynaptic motor reflexes play an important role in locomotion (locomotion reflexes), eating (nutritional reflexes), and protecting the body from its environment (protective reflexes). Examples of each of these types of reflex will be introduced below. In defining the characteristics of the extrinsic reflexes we should always bear in mind that even in the case of the monosynaptic stretch reflex the reflex response is not firmly coupled to the stimulus (in automaton-like fashion), but instead it can be modified by other excitatory and inhibitory influences acting simultaneously on the motoneuron. Thanks to the large number of neurons involved, it is much easier in a polysynaptic reflex arc to adapt the reflex response to the prevailing requirements of the body.

Examples of polysynaptic motor reflexes.   Figure 4-4A shows that the Ia fibers coming from the stretch receptors of the muscle spindles form not only monosynaptic excitatory synapses with homonymous motoneurons but also *inhibitory* synapses with *antagonistic motoneurons.* The inhibitory connection is made through an interneuron (shown in red in Fig. 4-4A). The inhibitory reflex arc of the Ia fibers on antagonistic motoneurons thus has *two* central synapses, one from the Ia fiber on the interneuron (excitatory synapse) and the other from the axon of the interneuron on the motoneuron (inhibitory synapse). It is the shortest known inhibitory reflex arc. This type of inhibition therefore is also called *direct inhibition.*

Most of the other excitatory and inhibitory afferents converging on the motoneurons from the peripheral receptors (from the muscles, joints, and skin) have more than one, often indeed very many, interneurons in their reflex arc. They are not disynaptic but polysynaptic. Let us consider two examples. Brushing a mother's nipple against the lips of her newborn child automatically triggers a sucking reaction. The same sucking reaction can be provoked by touching the lips with the tip of one's finger or by giving the child a pacifier (dummy). This clearly demonstrates the reflex character of this phenomenon. The *sucking reflex* is a *nutritional reflex*. The receptors of its polysynaptic reflex arc are touch-sensitive structures in the skin of the lips (mechanoreceptors). The effectors are the muscles of the lips, cheeks, tongue, throat, thorax, and diaphragm. The sucking reflex is thus a very complicated extrinsic reflex, and it should also be remembered that the sucking action has to be coordinated with normal respiration.

If a piece of filter paper soaked in acid is laid on the back of a decerebrate frog (with the cerebrum removed under anesthesia the frog can remain alive for many days and even weeks), then after a short latent period the frog will brush the piece of paper off with the nearest hind limb. This is an example of a *protective reflex*. In the case of this protective reflex, the (pain) receptors are located in the skin of the back while the musculature of the hind limb is the effector. This reflex is therefore also a polysynaptic extrinsic reflex.

Characteristics of polysynaptic reflexes.   The *cough reflex* serves to keep the respiratory passages free from blockages preventing inhalation and exhalation of air. The cough reflex is thus a typical *protective reflex*. The receptors are located in the mucous membrane of the windpipe (trachea) and its branches (bronchia). Stimulation of the mucous membrane receptors not only triggers the cough reflex but also generates conscious sensations so that we can compare the intensity of the stimulus and the size of the reflex response. We will therefore use this reflex to study the characteristic properties of polysynaptic reflexes.

You will almost certainly have noticed that a slight "tickling" or irritation in the throat does not make you cough immediately but only after a short time has elapsed. We can deduce from this that in the case of polysynaptic reflexes stimuli *subthreshold* to trigger the reflex can *summate* to a *suprathreshold* stimulus. This *summation* is a central phenomenon; that is, it takes place in the interneurons and the motoneurons of the reflex arc and not in the peripheral receptors. The subjective feelings of discomfort (tickling, irritation) experienced before the reflex is triggered are a clear sign that the receptors responsible for the reflex are already excited. We can state generally that in the case of polysynaptic reflexes initially subthreshold stimuli can summate to suprathreshold stimuli if they last long enough. With increasing stimulus intensity the time between the stimulus and the triggering of the reflex, that is, the *reflex time*, becomes shorter and shorter even when the stimuli are already above the threshold. We can generalize even more and say that in the case of the polysynaptic reflex the reflex time is dependent on the intensity of the stimulus; stronger stimuli cause the reflex to start sooner. (In contrast, in the monosynaptic stretch reflex the reflex time is relatively constant.) The shorter reflex time of the polysynaptic reflex with increasing stimulus intensity is a result of the more rapid suprathreshold excitation of the central neurons of the reflex arc which is brought about by the larger number of more intensely activated receptors. The shorter reflex time is caused mainly by temporal and spatial facilitation.

Coughing can range in intensity from simply clearing the throat to a long fit of choking coughs, again depending on the intensity of the stimulus. This increase in the *reflex response* with increasing intensity of the stimulus is also a typical characteristic of polysynaptic motor reflexes. In the process the reflex starts to affect previously uninvolved groups of muscles, a phenomenon called *spreading*. Obviously, with strong stimuli, neurons that were previously excited below the threshold now receive suprathreshold excitation. The *spreading* of the reflex is particularly easy to demonstrate in the case of coughing. When we simply clear our throats it is chiefly the muscles of the throat that are activated, while in the case of a choking cough the muscles of the chest, shoulders, abdomen, and diaphragm are involved.

Motor reflexes and autonomic polysynaptic reflexes. In the motor reflexes, for example, the locomotion, the nutritional, and the protective reflexes, the motoaxons form the efferent pathway of the reflex arc while the receptors are situated primarily in the skin, the muscles, the tendons, and the joints. There are also a large number of polysynaptic reflexes that likewise end at motoneurons but that originate in visceral receptors. The most obvious example is that of the respiratory reflexes that originate from stretch receptors of the lung and from chemoreceptors, and whose efferent pathways are formed by the motoaxons of the diaphragm and the respiratory muscles in the thorax. The neurons of the autonomic nervous system that lead to glands and smooth muscles are the efferent pathways for a large number of *autonomic* reflexes. We shall take a closer look at some examples of these in Chapter 8. At this point it is sufficient just to mention the key words "circulatory reflexes," "digestive reflexes," and "sexual reflexes."

The didactically expedient grouping and classifying of the polysynaptic reflexes should not blind us to the fact that there are many mixed types of polysynaptic reflexes and that each of the known "classifications" is in one way or another arbitrary. For example, the cough reflex is certainly a protective reflex, but it is not, in the strict sense, a motor reflex, because its receptors are situated in the mucous membrane of the trachea and the bronchia; they are thus visceroreceptors. Many of the complex reflexes, for example, the sexual reflexes, also simultaneously possess motor and autonomic efferent pathways. A further aspect, which can easily be overlooked if individual reflexes are considered in isolation, is that most motoneurons and interneurons are represented in a large number of reflex arcs. A motoaxon in the musculature of the throat will, for example, be involved in swallowing, sucking, coughing, sneezing, and respiratory reflexes; that is, it will offer the same final common pathway for a large number of reflex arcs.

Congenital and acquired reflexes. The reflexes we have considered so far all involve stereotyped reactions of the organism that are predetermined in the structural design of the CNS. They can be observed in practically the same form in all individuals of the same species. The neurons of these preformed reflex arcs are mostly situated in the phylogenetically older parts of the CNS, that is, in the spinal cord and the brain stem, even when the reflexes involved are highly complex (for example, protection reflex in decerebrate frog when acid is applied to its back). Each individual in addition has the ability to acquire reflex reactions so that his body can respond better and with less effort to the constantly changing situations in his environment. The reflex arcs of these acquired reflexes usually run in the higher sections of the CNS. The acquired reflexes (which can also be forgotten again) are distinguished from the stereotyped congenital reactions of the organism by a wide range of criteria. These criteria and classification systems will not be treated here, however.

Work through the next steps to check your new knowledge.

Q 4.9 Which of the following are nutritional reflexes and which are protective?
   a. Reflex governing secretion of tears.
   b. Reflex governing secretion of saliva.
   c. Corneal (eyelid closure) reflex.
   d. Sucking reflex.
   e. Sneezing reflex.
   f. Cough reflex.

Q 4.10 Which of the following are due to summation?
   a. The increase in the size of the reflex response with increasing intensity of the stimulus.

    b. The modification of the reflex response by influences simultaneously acting on the interneurons of the reflex arc.

    c. The shortening of the latent period between commencement of the stimulus and onset of the reflex with increasing stimulus intensity.

    d. The simultaneous inhibition of antagonistic motoneurons when homonymous motoneurons are excited by Ia fibers.

Q 4.11 How many central synapses are involved in the reflex arc of direct inhibition?

    a. None.

    b. One.

    c. Two.

    d. Three.

    e. Many.

Q 4.12 Which of the following central neuronal processes are involved in the spreading of polysynaptic motor reflexes?

    a. Direct inhibition.

    b. Temporal facilitation.

    c. Posttetanic potentiation.

    d. Occlusion.

    e. Spatial facilitation.

    f. None of these processes.

    g. All of these processes.

5

MUSCLES

By far the most extensively developed organ in the bodies of man and other vertebrates is that of the musculature, the "flesh." The muscles make up 40 to 50 percent of the total body weight. Their main function is to contract in order to develop force. They are also, among other things, important for the thermal regulation of the body, but the heat-producing role of the musculature will not be discussed here in connection with the neurophysiological features.

Man can make an impact on his environment only by utilizing his muscles. This is true not just for physical work but for intellectual activity as well, for both writing and speaking require a finely tuned interplay between muscles. One could regard the nervous system, perhaps a little one-sidedly, as an organ that responds to the stimuli acting on the organism by producing corresponding muscle contractions. This means that the muscle is a highly important subject for the neurophysiologist. Furthermore, the modus operandi of the muscle cells is better known than that of most other types of cells. The morphology and the chemical components and reactions as well as the physiological functions of muscle cells have been very extensively researched, and in recent years the various approaches have been combined into a unified theory of muscle contraction. When discussing the function of muscles, we must therefore pay particular attention to their structure and chemical composition.

5.1 Contraction of the Muscle

The most important part of the musculature, the *skeletal muscles*, is divided into individual muscles, such as those shown in Fig. 5-3 from the dorsal part of the upper arm. Such a muscle is an elongated "bundle of tissue" terminating at both ends in cord-like *tendons*. The muscle is connected through the tendons with the bones, the "skeleton," and can thus act on the latter. In order to study its function, the muscle is usually isolated. This is easily achieved by severing the tendons. The muscle then can be suitably attached by way of the tendon stumps in a test bath (see Fig. 5-1). The reactions of such a muscle specimen to excitation of its fibers will now be discussed.

Isotonic and isometric contraction. If a muscle is stimulated by impulses in the motor nerve (see page 66) or by direct suprathreshold depolarization of its fibers, then it *contracts*; that is, it tries to become shorter and, as a result, exerts a pull on its points of attachment. Whether or not shortening of the muscle occurs during contraction depends on whether its attachment points are able to yield. It is therefore necessary to define the way in which the muscle is fixed when its contraction is measured. It is customary to measure contraction in one of two different ways:

1.   The contraction can be measured by firmly attaching the muscle at one end and hanging a *movable but constant load* on the other end (Fig. 5-1A). The shortening of the muscle measured under these constant load conditions is called *isotonic contraction*.

2.   The contraction can also be measured by firmly clamping both ends of the muscle so that they cannot move and incorporating a force meter at one end which does not vary in length under load (Fig. 5-1B).

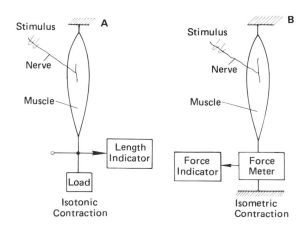

Fig. 5-1.   Measurement of contraction. *A*: Measurement of isotonic contraction. The muscle is attached at one end and lifts a constant load. The change in length of the muscle is recorded. *B*: Measurement of isometric contraction. The muscle is attached at both ends and thus has a constant length. The changes in force exerted by the muscle at its points of attachment are recorded.

The change in force measured while the *length of the muscle remains constant* is called *isometric contraction.*

When the muscles contract naturally, the contraction is rarely fully isotonic or fully isometric. For example, when a bucket of water is raised by the arm, the arm undergoes "isotonic shortening," but, because of the change in the angular configuration of the bones when the arm is bent, the load on the individual muscles in the arm does not remain fully constant. Approximately isometric conditions exist, for example, when the trunk is stabilized by simultaneous contraction of the dorsal and the abdominal muscles, for example, when one "stands at attention."

Time course of individual contraction. When a muscle is excited by a single stimulus, then it contracts briefly, or twitches. Under isotonic conditions this single contraction is recorded as transitory shortening of the muscle; under isometric conditions it is recorded as a transitory increase in force. A typical time course of *isometric contraction* in a muscle of a warm-blooded animal is shown in Fig. 5-2. The contraction is triggered by the action potential shown in the top half of the figure, and it begins *a few milliseconds* after the upstroke of the action potential. The force exerted reaches its maximum in about 80 msec and returns somewhat more slowly to the resting value. We can distinguish, therefore, between a *rising phase* and a *relaxation phase* of the contraction. In the case of isotonic contraction the time

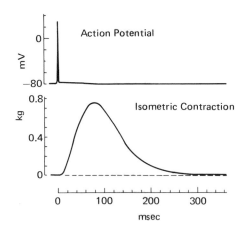

Fig. 5-2. Action potential and muscle contraction. Time course of the action potential and of the subsequent contraction of a human thumb muscle (adductor pollicis). The contraction commences about 2 msec after the upstroke of the action potential and reaches its maximum only after 100 msec.

course of the change in length is quite similar to the time course of force shown in Fig. 5-2. If we compare the time course of contraction with the duration of the action potential it is obvious that the contraction takes place much more slowly. The action potential is almost finished before the start of the contraction it triggers. The contraction of the muscle is thus about 100 times slower than the action potential.

However, the duration of the muscle contraction is less uniform than the duration of the action potential in the various muscles. The contraction curve for a thumb muscle shown in Fig. 5-2 is an example of a *"fast"* muscle as found in warm-blooded animals. These animals also have *slow* muscles that take 200 msec to attain their maximum contraction, and in low-temperature muscles of cold-blooded animals the rising phase of contraction can last several seconds.

Fine structure of the skeletal muscles.   The mechanism of muscle contraction can be more accurately explained only if the fine structure of the muscle fiber is known. This fine structure is illustrated in Fig. 5-3. The upper arm muscle shown in Fig. 5-3A is composed of bundles of fibers (Fig. 5-3B) that are still easily visible to the naked eye (think of the "fibers" in boiled beef). The individual *muscle fibers* of the bundle (Fig. 5-3C) are cells measuring several to many centimeters in length and 10 to 100 μ in diameter. The muscle fibers mostly run through the entire length of the muscle and terminate at both ends in the connective tissue tendons. The muscle fibers contain high concentrations of contractile protein structures that are arranged in fiber form in the longitudinal direction of the muscle cell and are called *myofibrils* (Fig. 5-3C).

When viewed under the microscope, the muscle fibers exhibit a characteristic *cross striation*. The striated pattern is produced by the structures running the length of the fibers, the myofibrils, which are themselves cross striated (Fig. 5-3D) and arranged in strict side-by-side configuration in the fiber. The striation of the adjacent myofibrils is caused by the fact that they contain strongly birefringent (anisotropic) and weakly birefringent (isotropic) parts in regularly alternating sequence. In transmitted light the strongly birefringent striations are darker than the weakly birefringent ones. Accordingly, as shown in Fig. 5-3D, they are termed *A bands* and *I bands*. A thin dark strip is located in the middle of the I band. This is called the Z disc. The distance between two Z discs is the smallest, about 2 μ long, functional unit of the myofibril and is called the *sarcomere*.

The fine structure of the sarcomere can be resolved further with an electron microscope (Fig. 5-3E-I). As Fig. 5-3E shows, the Z disc links adjacent *thin myofilaments*. In the central section of the sarcomere

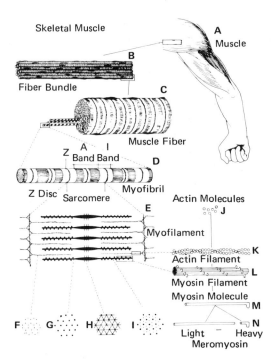

Fig. 5-3. Fine structure of skeletal muscle. Diagrams of muscular structure from the complete muscle through muscle fibers, myofibrils, and
myofilaments to the molecular structure of the contractile proteins. See text
for detailed description. (Redrawn from Bloom and Fawcett, A *Textbook of
Histology, Saunders, Philadelphia, 1969.*)

thick myofilaments are situated between the thin myofilaments. The
cross sections in Fig. 5-3F to I show that the thin and the thick myofilaments are arranged in strictly ordered arrays in a manner reminiscent of crystal structures. Using chemical methods it has been
shown that the thin myofilaments consist of the protein *actin* (Fig. 5-3
J-K) and the thick myofilaments consist of other elongated protein
molecules, namely, *myosin* (Fig. 5-3 *L–N*). Thus the I bands of the
myofibrils consist mainly of the protein actin, and the A bands in the
central portion consist entirely of the protein myosin. In the lateral
sections of the A band both actin and myosin are present.

**Displacement of the actin and the myosin filaments during con-
traction.** The chemical and physical processes on which contraction
is based become clear when one observes the behavior of the structural elements of the muscle, as illustrated in Fig. 5-3, during contraction. If the muscle can shorten, for example, in the case of isotonic

contraction, the width of the *A bands remains constant* while the *I bands become narrower*. The birefringence in the A band is caused by the presence of the myosin filaments. If the width of the A bands remains constant during contraction, the length of the myosin filaments must also stay constant.

The I band becomes narrower during isotonic contraction. Nevertheless, electron microscope images reveal that the actin filaments, which are the sole constituents of the I band, stay the same length during contraction. Since the lengths of the actin and the myosin filaments do not change, the length of the sarcomere can only decrease during contraction as a result of the *filaments sliding past each other* (sliding-filament theory). The I band is thus narrowed because the myosin filaments within it slide between the actin filaments.

The movement of the myosin and the actin filaments during contraction is illustrated in Fig. 5-4, which shows diagrams of the sarcomere at the start and the peak of contraction. During contraction (from *A* to *B*) the sarcomere becomes shorter, and the distance between the Z discs becomes smaller because the myosin and the actin filaments slide past each other. The ends of the myosin filaments approach the Z discs, and the I bands consequently become narrower

Molecular mechanism of contraction. What forces bring about the displacement of the myofilaments during contraction? In Fig. 5-4 oblique strokes have been drawn between the actin and the myosin filaments, starting from the myosin filaments. These strokes are supposed to represent bridges, groups of molecules, which produce chemical bonds between myosin and actin. When a bond is formed in

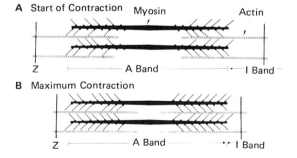

Fig. 5-4. Mechanism of contraction. Diagram of the arrangement of the myosin and the actin filaments in a sarcomere (from Z to Z) and of the bridges existing between these filaments. It is assumed that the bridges can shorten, and as a result the actin filaments slide between the myosin filaments. *A:* Condition at the start of contraction. *B:* Condition at maximum contraction; the sarcomere has become shorter.

the manner indicated in Fig. 5-4, the individual bridges *shorten* and draw the actin filaments between the myosin filaments. After shortening is complete, the bridge is broken once more, and the cycle can start over again. In other words, a new bridge forms between the actin and the myosin filaments which have just been displaced, the bridge shortens itself, and so on as before.

The bridges, which by shortening bring about the relative displacement of the actin and the myosin filaments, and thus the contraction of the muscle, originate at the thickened end of the myosin molecule. Figure 5-3L shows that the myosin filament is built up of a staggered configuration of adjacent myosin molecules (Fig. 5-3M). The thickened ends of the myosin molecules are distributed regularly along the filament. This thick portion of the myosin is called "heavy meromyosin" (Fig. 5-3N). On the one hand, the heavy meromyosin is a substance that can form chemical bonds with the actin, but on the other hand, it is an enzyme that *splits off* a phosphate from the *adenosine triphosphate* (ATP) in the cell, releasing energy in the process. Part of this energy is used to shorten the bridges between myosin and actin, and some is given off as heat. Muscular contraction is thus caused by the formation of complexes of *myosin, actin, and ATP*, with ATP being split and the bridges between myosin and actin becoming shorter.

The reaction of myosin, actin, and ATP, on which muscular contraction is based, can take place only when Ca^{++} *ions* are present in the cell in a free concentration of approximately 10^{-5} M. In addition, contraction requires the presence of Mg^{++} ions. In the relaxed muscle the Ca^{++} concentration is 10^{-8} M, and consequently the reaction between myosin, actin, and ATP cannot take place. The cell possesses a mechanism by which the Ca^{++} concentration can be raised to 10^{-5} M, permitting the reaction of actin, myosin, and ATP, and thereby initiating contraction. At the molecular level, therefore, contraction is controlled by the Ca^{++} concentration. This process is discussed in detail in Sec. 5.3.

Besides supplying the energy for muscular contraction, ATP has another effect on the contractile system. The bridge between myosin and actin will break down again only in the presence of ATP at the end of contraction when the intracellular Ca^{++} concentration drops to 10^{-8} M. This action of ATP is known as the *plasticizer effect*. When the ATP concentration in a muscle drops following a reduction in the supply of energy, the muscle cannot relax; it remains "hard" or rigid. After death, too, the ATP concentration in the muscle drops, the plasticizer effect of the ATP on the myosin-actin complex is removed, and rigor mortis sets in.

Cardiac muscles and smooth muscles. In this section we have taken a detailed look at the fine structure and the contraction mechanism of skeletal muscle fibers. Apart from this quantitatively predominant type of muscle there are also the cardiac muscles and the smooth muscles to consider. The latter consist of fibers shorter and thinner than those of the skeletal muscles, and these fibers are interconnected in reticular fashion. The smooth muscle fibers, like the skeletal muscle system, contain myofibrils, but the latter are neither as densely packaged nor as regularly arranged as in the skeletal muscles. Therefore, no cross striation is visible in the *smooth muscles*. The contraction of the myofibrils in the smooth musculature occurs in exactly the same way as in the skeletal muscle fibers. Since the action potentials in smooth muscle are propagated differently from those in skeletal muscle, the time course of contraction in smooth muscles is on the whole slower than in the skeletal muscle system. This fact will be examined in greater detail in Chapter 8.

As regards structure and time course of contraction, the *cardiac muscles* constitute a transitional form between skeletal and smooth muscles. However, the contraction mechanism in cardiac muscles is the same as in skeletal muscles.

The following questions will check how far you have assimilated the information given in this chapter.

Q 5.1 Draw a sketch showing how a muscle fibril is composed of thick and thin myofilaments and illustrating how the filaments are connected to the Z discs. Indicate in your sketch the length of the sarcomere and insert the chemical names of the protein elements that make up the myofilaments.

Q 5.2 During isotonic contraction the
    a. contraction force varies while the length of the muscle remains constant.
    b. length of the muscle changes while the load on the muscle remains constant.
    c. length of the sarcomere remains constant.
    d. Sarcomere becomes shorter.
    e. anisotropic and the isotropic bands become shorter.
    f. isotropic bands become shorter and the anisotropic bands remain constant.
    g. anisotropic bands become shorter and the isotropic bands remain constant.
    (More than one of the above answers is correct.)

Q 5.3 Indicating the time scale, sketch the time course of isometric contraction in a muscle from a warm-blooded animal.

Q 5.4 Which four substances, apart from Mg^{++} ions, take part in the chemical reaction on which contraction is based or must be present in adequate concentration during the reaction? Underline the substance that supplies the energy for the contraction.

1. . . . .
2. . . . .
3. . . . .
4. . . . .

5.2 Dependence of Muscle Contraction on Fiber Length and Velocity of Contraction

In the preceding section the mechanism of contraction of the muscle fiber was described. During muscular contraction the actin filaments are drawn between the myosin filaments. However, the extent to which this fundamental process manifests itself as force developed at the tendons and the extent to which the muscle becomes shorter both depend on the circumstances accompanying the muscular contraction. The strongest influence is exerted on the contraction by the length of the fibers at the start of contraction, the amount of prestretching, as well as the rate at which the contractile elements become shorter. Since these parameters are also of great importance *in vivo* for the course of the contraction and since they are partly responsible for controlling the development of force, they will now be discussed in detail.

The length-tension curve.   Muscles, or also isolated muscle fibers, kept at their "resting length" exert no force at their points of attachment. If one end of the muscle is pulled, the muscle is stretched. If the force necessary to produce stretching is plotted against the muscle length, the *length-tension* curve shown in Fig. 5-5 (resting) is obtained. The force increases exponentially with length starting from zero at the resting length, l_0. The muscle is not damaged by being stretched to about 1.8 times its resting length, but any additional stretching would tear the muscle fibers.

When the muscle is stretched, elongation first occurs in the sarcomere as the actin and the myosin filaments slide past each other (see Fig. 5-4). When this happens the I bands become broader and the A bands remain unchanged. Besides the elongation in the contractile elements, the sarcomeres, there is also elongation in the passive *elastic elements* during stretching of the muscle. These passive elastic elements are mainly the tendons on which the muscle terminates. As will be discussed further below, the stretching of the passive elastic elements is very important for the dynamics of muscular contraction.

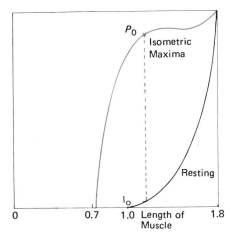

Fig. 5-5. Length-tension curve and isometric maxima. Dependence of force on muscle length in the resting muscle. Length-tension curve (black) and curve of isometric maxima (red). l_0 is the resting length of the muscle. Multiples of l_0 are plotted along the abscissa. P_0 is the maximum additional isometric force, that is, the maximum increase in force during an isometric contraction.

The curve of the isometric maxima. The amount of prestretching of the muscle is important not only with regard to the resting tension of the muscle, but it also determines the amount of force developed by a muscle during contraction. For example, if isometric contractions are measured by the procedure illustrated in Fig. 5-1, the length of the muscle can be set before each contraction by moving the points of attachment to the desired positions. When the muscle is made to contract from various initial lengths, the force increases in each case above the initial tension to the *"isometric maximum."* The curve of the isometric maxima is drawn in red in Fig. 5-5. The force developed beyond the resting tension for a given muscle length is the difference between the curve of the isometric maxima and the length-tension curve.

The muscle develops its maximum force (P_0) at around the resting length, l_0. The force developed is very much reduced if the muscle is shorter than the resting length, l_0, when contraction begins. The point of intersection of the red curve with the abscissa in Fig. 5-5 denotes the shortest length at which the muscle can still just develop force. Thus, in the case of *isotonic* contraction, the muscle could shorten at the most to *about 70 percent of the resting length l_0.* The force developed during isometric contraction also declines when the muscle is stretched far beyond the resting length. At approximately 1.8 times the resting length the curves in Fig. 5-5 run together, and at the point where they meet, the muscle develops *no more force* during contraction. Consequently, the muscle can develop force only in the range from 70 percent resting length to 180 percent resting length.

The dependence of the contractile force on the amount of *prestretching* can be explained by the *arrangement of the myofilaments* in the sarcomere. In Fig. 5-6 the isometrically developed force is shown for a sarcomere as a function of the sarcomere length. To the right of the curve are shown the various arrangements of the myosin and the actin filaments in the sarcomere, as determined by electron microscopy, for various sarcomere lengths (A to E). At maximum prestretching (A) the filaments no longer overlap, and no bridges can form between them nor can contractile force be developed. Given less prestretching (between A and B) the overlapping of the myofilaments increases, and the amount of contractile force developed increases proportionately. The optimum contractile force is attained (between B and C) when bridges can be formed to the actin along the entire length of the myosin filament.

At muscle lengths shorter than the resting length (C to E) the contractile force declines rapidly because the actin filaments are drawn in so far between the myosin filaments that they interfere with

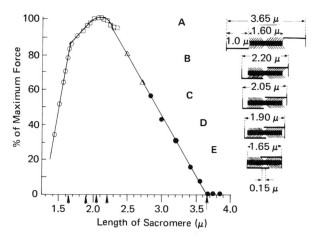

Fig. 5-6. Maximum isometric force developed at various sarcomere lengths. In the graph the maximum additional isometric force is plotted as a function of the sarcomere length. On the right, in A to E, is shown the overlapping of the actin and the myosin filaments for sarcomere lengths from 3.65 to 1.65 μ. The lengths A to E are also shown at the corresponding points along the abscissa of the graph. The dependence of the force developed on the length of the sarcomere can be deduced from diagrams A to E. See text for more details. (From Ruch and Patton, *Physiology and Biophysics*, Saunders, Philadelphia, 1965.)

each other at the center, or the Z discs run up against the myo-filaments (*E*). The dependence of contractile force on the amount of prestretching can thus be explained quantitatively by the degree of overlap between the myosin and the actin filaments. The chemical reaction on which contraction is based can only take place when the actin and the myosin filaments are closely adjacent. The contractile force is proportional to the number of actin and myosin molecules reacting with each other per unit time.

Force and velocity of contraction. The dependence of the contractile force on the amount of prestretching has been explained in terms of the structure of the contractile apparatus. Similarly, the influence exerted by the velocity of shortening on the amount of force developed can also be attributed to the characteristics of the contractile apparatus.

Consider some everyday examples of muscular function in our own bodies. We can exert maximum force with our muscles only if they do not shorten in the process or if the shortening is only slight, for example, when we press or push against something. In contrast, we can carry out rapid movements only when the muscles are very lightly loaded, or in other words, when the musculature is supple, for example, when we throw a stone or play the piano.

Figure 5-7 shows the connection between the maximum velocity of shortening and the force developed by an isolated arm muscle.

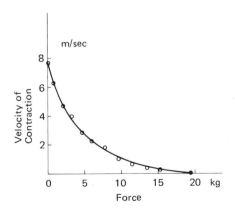

Fig. 5-7. Velocity of contraction of a muscle as a function of the force exerted. The abscissa values correspond to the loading of the muscle during isotonic contraction; the ordinate values give the maximum velocity of shortening of the muscle. The interpolated curve is a segment of a hyperbola. (From Wilkie, *J. Physiol.* **110**, 249, 1949.)

Without becoming shorter, this muscle can exert a force of 19 kg. As the load decreases, however, it contracts at an increasingly rapid rate, and at load zero a velocity of contraction of almost 8 m/sec is attained. A similar relationship between force and velocity of shortening is found in all muscles. The decrease in contractile force with increasing velocity of shortening can be explained quantitatively in terms of the contraction mechanism of the myosin and the actin filaments that slide past each other. The force developed by the muscle is in fact proportional to the number of bridges that form between the myosin and the actin filaments per unit time (see Fig. 5-6). As the myosin and the actin filaments slide faster past each other during contraction, the number of bridges that can be formed per unit time between the filaments decreases. The contractile force thus declines with the velocity of shortening.

The decrease in the velocity of shortening with increasing load is usually measured in the case of *isotonic* contraction, that is, when the muscle shortens under constant load. However, the velocity of contraction also has an effect in the case of isometric contraction when no actual shortening occurs. At the level of the contractile unit, the sarcomere, there are, in fact, *no strictly isometric contractions.* During isometric contraction of the muscle its elastic elements, particularly the tendons, are stretched. As a result, even during isometric contraction, the sarcomeres can shorten, and the myosin and the actin filaments can slide past each other. This displacement of the myofibrils reduces the amount of force that can be developed during contraction. Thus the maximum muscle force for zero velocity of shortening of the sarcomeres is not reached by isometric contraction either. This fact is a precondition for a functionally very important mechanism: summation of individual muscular contractions. The process of summation will now be examined in more detail.

Summation of individual contractions (twitches); tetanus. Figure 5-8 *A* shows a single isometric contraction (twitch) in a rapid-acting muscle of a warm-blooded animal. This contraction rises in less than 50 msec to its maximum, and it drops again somewhat more slowly (see also Fig. 5-2). If the muscle is stimulated again before it has fully relaxed, then the next contraction starts from a higher initial tension, and it attains a higher maximum force than the first contraction (Fig. 5-8*B*). This event is called *summation.*

In the body, muscles are usually stimulated by a series of action potentials. If the time between the action potentials is shorter than the overall duration of contraction, that is, if the frequency of the action potentials is greater than 5 to 10/sec, then, as shown in Fig. 5-8*B* to *E,*

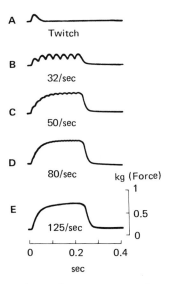

Fig. 5-8. Summation of twitches up to complete tetanus. Isometrically measured contractions of a rapid muscle in a warm-blooded animal (flexor hallucis longus of the cat). *A*: Twitch. *B* to *E*: Series of contractions generated by stimuli having the frequencies as shown under the individual curves. In *C* and *D* incomplete tetanus, and in *E* complete tetanus is attained. (From Buller and Lewis, *J. Physiol.*, **176**, 337, 1965.)

summation occurs for each new contraction. However, summation of the individual contractions is *not linear*. Figure 5-8*B* to *D* shows clearly that the increase in contractile force per individual contraction decreases with the number of stimuli within the series. If the series of stimuli is long enough, then, after a certain number of stimuli, there is absolutely no further increase in contractile force during the individual contractions. The contraction reaches a plateau at which the contractile force fluctuates slightly.

A series of contractions that, through summation of the individual contractions, attains a more or less steady and maintained force is called a *tetanus* or tetanic contraction. In Fig. 5-8*C* to *E* a tetanus is measured at stimulus frequencies from 50 to 125/sec. But a completely uniform force without visible fluctuation occurs only at the maximum stimulus frequency of 125/sec. This condition is called *fused (complete) tetanus*. At lower stimulus frequencies the force fluctuates approximately in time with the stimuli; that is, the tetanus is *unfused*. The fused tetanus attained at high stimulus frequency by summation of the individual contractions is the *maximum force* the muscle can generate for that particular amount of prestretching. This force is two to five times greater than that attained during a single contraction.

Mechanism of summation. The maximum possible force of which a muscle is capable is not developed during a single contraction. This might lead one to suppose that the contractile system is not fully activated during a single twitch and that the chemical reactions on which contraction is based do not take place to the full extent. However, this is not the case. Using methods that will not be discussed in further detail here, it has been shown that even during the single contraction the contractile system is fully activated for a short time; that is, the myosin-actin reaction takes place completely with adenosine triphosphate being split. Nevertheless, only part of the tetanic force is developed at the tendons during a twitch because during this phase the sarcomeres become shorter. As discussed above, the same is also true for isometric contractions, for with increasing force the elastic elements become longer. Thus, during the rising phase of isometric twitches the sarcomeres *shorten* at a certain rate, and this *reduces* the force developed (see Fig. 5-7).

If the muscle fiber is restimulated before a twitch is complete, the sarcomeres will still be shortened from the first contraction. Therefore they can shorten less during the second contraction than during the first, and as a result greater force will be developed during the second contraction and at a slower velocity of shortening. This mechanism is called *summation*. Summation thus is caused not by a stronger reaction of the contractile system but by prestretching of the elastic elements by the preceding contraction. If the muscle is stimulated at a sufficiently high frequency, *tetanic* contractions are generated. In the process, by repetitive activation of the contractile system, the sarcomeres become so short that the tensile force taken up by the elastic elements equals the maximum contractile force. In this state of equilibrium the sarcomeres no longer change their lengths, and at *zero velocity of shortening* the *maximum contractile force* is fully measurable at the tendons.

The following questions will check whether you remember what you have learned in this chapter.

Q 5.5 Which of the following statements correctly apply to the curve of the isometric maxima? (Check off the correct answers.)
   a. The maximum force is developed at approximately half the resting length.
   b. The maximum force is developed at the muscle length at which the maximum overlapping of myosin and actin filaments occurs during contraction.
   c. The maximum force is developed at the resting length.
   d. The maximum force is developed at the muscle length at which myosin and actin filaments overlap least during contraction.

    e. The overlapping of the myosin and actin filaments is optimum
       for contraction at the point of intersection of the curve of the
       isometric maxima and the length-tension curve.

Q 5.6 The contractile force of the muscle decreases with the velocity of
    shortening because
    a. there is an insufficient supply of adenosine triphosphate
       available at high velocity of shortening.
    b. the work performed increases in proportion to the velocity of
       shortening.
    c. the number of bridges existing per unit time between the
       myosin and the actin filaments decreases with the velocity of
       shortening.
    d. the number of bridges existing per unit time between the
       myosin and the actin filaments increases with the velocity of
       shortening.

Q 5.7 Which of the following statements apply in the case of the sum-
    mation of muscle contractions?
    a. Muscle contractions are summated when the second stimulus
       occurs in the refractory phase of the first stimulus.
    b. Muscle contractions are summated when the second contrac-
       tion is triggered before the first contraction has died away.
    c. Through summation of muscle contractions a force is gener-
       ated which is proportional to the number of summated con-
       tractions.

Q 5.8 Muscle contractions of individual fibers can be summated be-
    cause
    a. not all the myofibrils are activated for each contraction.
    b. the contractile system is not supplied with sufficient ATP
       during a contraction.
    c. in the case of a twitch the sarcomeres still continue to shorten
       throughout the state of maximum activation of the contractile
       system.
    d. in the case of a twitch, the state of maximum activation of the
       contractile system does not last long enough to permit max-
       imum shortening of the sarcomeres.

5.3 Electromechanical Coupling

Humans and animals can move only with the aid of their muscles
and can make an impact on their environment only if the muscle
contractions can be controlled exactly. Control is exerted by the motor
nervous system, which, through activation of the motor nerves, elicits
end-plate potentials in the muscle fibers (see Chapter 3). These end-
plate potentials trigger action potentials that are conducted along the

muscle fibers. Excitation of the membrane is followed by contraction of the fiber. A change in the membrane potential thus controls the reaction of the contractile proteins of the muscle. This process is called *electromechanical coupling* and will be studied in more detail in this section.

Dependence of contractile force on membrane potential. The phenomenon of electromechanical coupling can be studied particularly well by triggering contraction by means of sudden enforced changes in the membrane potential to any arbitrary value (voltage clamp; see page 41). The dependence of contractile force on membrane potential as measured in this way is shown in Fig. 5-9. If, starting from the resting potential, the muscle fiber is depolarized to −55 mV, then no contraction occurs. The *mechanical threshold* is crossed at slightly stronger depolarizations from −50 mV on, and the muscle contracts. However, unlike the excitation of the membrane the contraction does not obey the all-or-nothing law. In the range between −50 and −20 mV the contractile force increases approximately in proportion to the depolarization. In this potential range the extent of the contraction is *controllable* by the depolarization. Once the depolarization attains −20 mV or more positive values, no further changes occur in the contractile force even if depolarization continues. In this *saturation range* of depolarization the maximum force is thus developed independently of the membrane potential.

At its peak, the *action potential* in the muscle fiber reaches a potential more positive than −20 mV (see Fig. 2-10); therefore it *fully*

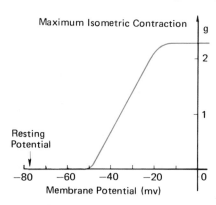

Fig. 5-9. Dependence of contractile force on membrane potential. The muscle develops force only when the potential crosses the mechanical threshold at about −50 mV. Between −50 and −20 mV the force is approximately proportional to the depolarization, but it barely increases at depolarizations above −20 mV.

activates the contractile system for a short time. Admittedly, this activation of the contractile system by an action potential does not last long enough for the maximum isometric force to be measurable (see page 130).

Because of the all-or-nothing character of the *action potential*, gradation of the contraction by graduated depolarization is not effective in the case of skeletal muscle fibers. Since every action potential in a muscle fiber follows the same course, the contractile system is always activated to the same extent and for the same length of time. In contrast to the skeletal muscles, however, the smooth musculature can be depolarized to various potentials by synaptic potentials or by stretching (see page 242). In these muscles, for example, the amount of force generated is also controlled by the degree of depolarization of the fiber membrane.

Function of the endoplasmic reticulum. The *control* of the development of force by the amount of depolarization is a *very rapid* process. The development of force starts to increase steeply 1 to 2 msec after the peak of the action potential (see Fig. 5-2), and the contractile system is fully activated within a few milliseconds. This rapid coupling between membrane depolarization and contraction of the intracellular myofibrils cannot be brought about by diffusion of a substance from the membrane to the myofibrils because such diffusion would take more than 1 to 2 msec. Thus electromechanical coupling in the skeletal muscles is not the result of certain substances flowing into the cell during excitation. Instead, the membrane depolarization has to be transmitted to the interior of the cell by special processes.

A special structural complex has been developed in the case of the relatively thick skeletal muscle fibers for the rapid coupling of membrane depolarization and contraction. This system is called the *endoplasmic reticulum*. It comprises two systems of hollow spaces or "tubes" within the muscle fibers. These will be discussed in conjunction with Fig. 5-10. To the right in Fig. 5-10 is the cell membrane, called here the sarcolemma. At regular intervals thin tubes, the transverse tubuli, invaginate into this outer cell membrane. These tubes run deeply into the fiber and sometimes transverse it completely at the level of the Z discs. Since the transverse tubuli are invaginations of the outer membrane, their interior is directly connected with the extracellular space.

A second tubular system, the *sarcoplasmic reticulum*, borders on the transverse tubuli (see Fig. 5-10). This second system runs at right angles to the transverse tubuli and parallel to the myofilaments of the

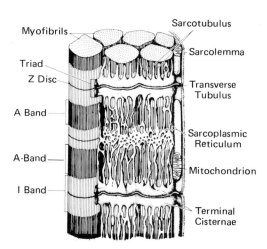

Fig. 5-10. Endoplasmic reticulum of a skeletal muscle fiber. Sketch of the fine structure of part of a muscle fiber based on an electron microscope image. At the right-hand side of the sketch the outer cell membrane is labeled sarcolemma. Transverse tubuli invaginate into the membrane and run across the fiber at the level of the Z discs. Between the Z discs and parallel to the myofibrils runs the sarcoplasmic reticulum, which abuts on the transverse tubuli with sacculate formations known as the terminal cisternae. A cross section through a transverse tubulus and abutting terminal cisternae reveals a configuration known as a triad (top left). (From Bloom and Fawcett, *A Textbook of Histology*, Saunders, Philadelphia, 1969.)

sarcomere. It is thus longitudinally aligned. The sarcoplasmic reticulum forms a network of hollow spaces from Z discs to Z discs along the myofibrils of each sarcomere. Where the sarcoplasmic reticulum abuts the transverse tubuli, it expands into terminal cisternae. A cross section through this region reveals a characteristic configuration of one thin tube accompanied on two sides by two thick tubes. This configuration is called a triad (see Fig. 5-10, left). It is clear from the figure that the transverse tubuli and the sarcoplasmic reticulum do not form a common system of hollow spaces, but instead are only in close contact with one another.

Function of the transverse tubuli. The transverse tubuli are invaginations of the outer cell membrane, and as such they extend the membrane into the interior of the cell and also enclose extracellular space. As a result, excitation of the outer cell membrane can be propagated in the transverse tubuli, and electrotonic depolarizations of the outer cell membrane can also be propagated via the transverse tubuli into the interior of the cell. The transverse tubuli can thus *rapidly conduct depolarizations of the outer membrane into the interior of the cell.* They permit rapid activation of the contractile system in the interior of the cell even in the case of large diameter fibers. The transverse tubuli are therefore particularly well developed in thick muscle fibers.

The role of the transverse tubuli in electromechanical coupling can be demonstrated by an elegant experiment. If, by applying a fine pipette against the cell membrane, only the mouth of a single tube is depolarized, the half sarcomeres on either side of the associated Z disc undergo local contraction. The extent of this contraction depends on the magnitude of the depolarizing current. The system of transverse tubuli associated with a Z disc thus controls the contraction in the half sarcomeres on either side of the Z disc.

Control of intracellular Ca^{++} concentration by the sarcoplasmic reticulum. But how does the system of transverse tubuli control contraction? In the discussion of the molecular mechanism of contraction it was stated that the Ca^{++} concentration in the intracellular space controls the reactions of the contractile proteins (see page 122). Myosin and actin can only link up, with adenosine triphosphate being broken down, if the Ca^{++} concentration reaches 10^{-5} M. The endoplasmic reticulum exercises control on contraction by bringing about rapid changes in the intracellular Ca^{++} concentration.

The *resting muscle fiber* has a very *low* Ca^{++} concentration of about 10^{-8} M. During *contraction* the concentration *increases* to about 10^{-5} M. These changes in the intracellular Ca^{++} concentration can be elegantly demonstrated by injecting a luminescent dye such as aequorin into a muscle fiber. The light emission of this dye is strongly dependent on the Ca^{++} concentration. When such a muscle fiber is depolarized, the light emission increases rapidly to a value corresponding to 10^{-5} M Ca^{++}. Then the light emission and thus also the free Ca^{++} concentration rapidly decline again.

What is the source of the Ca^{++} ions that increase the free Ca^{++} concentration in the intracellular space rapidly to 1,000 times the resting value following depolarization? A very high concentration of Ca^{++} ions was detected in the relaxed muscle in the terminal cisternae of the *sarcoplasmic reticulum*, close to the transverse tubuli (see Fig. 5-10). It is assumed that once the transverse tubuli have been depolarized they act in some as yet unknown way to cause an increase in membrane conductance for Ca^{++} ions in the *sarcoplasmic reticulum*. Because of the high concentration gradient *Ca^{++} ions then flow out* of the sarcoplasmic reticulum into the intracellular space. This raises the Ca^{++} concentration and permits the contraction-inducing reaction of myosin, actin, and adenosine triphosphate to take place. Electro-mechanical coupling is thus effected by controlling the Ca^{++} concentration. The various steps in the coupling process are shown once more in diagrammatic form in Fig. 5-11A. The depolarization of the cell membrane is conducted by the transverse tubuli to the interior of the cell. This depolarization causes the sarcoplasmic reticulum to release Ca^{++} ions. The Ca^{++} ions diffuse to the adjacent myofilaments where they make possible the chemical reactions that lead to contraction.

Once depolarization has come to an end, the intracellular Ca^{++} concentration drops very quickly and *relaxation* commences. The rapid drop in the intracellular Ca^{++} concentration is not due merely to the fact that the sarcoplasmic reticulum stops releasing Ca^{++}. Instead, the sarcoplasmic reticulum picks up Ca^{++} ions actively from the interior of the cell. An ion pump is situated in the membrane of the sarcoplasmic reticulum. By using metabolic energy, this pump transports Ca^{++} against the concentration gradient into the sarcoplasmic reticulum. The Ca^{++} pump of the *sarcoplasmic reticulum* operates very similarly as the Na^+ pump in the membrane of the nerve and the muscle fibers (see page 31) and other cells. By means of this Ca^{++}

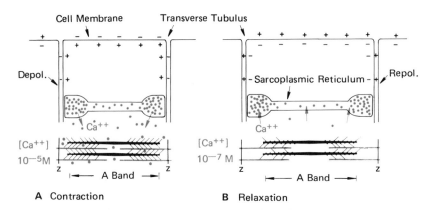

A Contraction   **B** Relaxation

Fig. 5-11. Electromechanical coupling. Diagram of the cell membrane showing the transverse tubuli with a portion of the sarcoplasmic reticulum between them and a sarcomere. The red dots denote Ca^{++} ions that are present in high concentration in the sarcoplasmic reticulum. During contraction in *A* the membrane of the sarcoplasmic reticulum becomes permeable to Ca^{++} ions following depolarization of the transverse tubuli. The Ca^{++} ions flow out and enable the myofilaments to contract. During muscular relaxation in *B* the transverse tubuli are repolarized, the Ca^{++} efflux from the sarcoplasmic reticulum therefore ceases, and the reticulum actively pumps Ca^{++} from the intracellular space. Contraction ceases when the intracellular concentration of free Ca^{++} is low.

pump the free Ca^{++} concentration in the intracellular space is maintained at a very low level (10^{-8} M) under resting conditions, and the sarcoplasmic reticulum can store Ca^{++} in high concentrations. The pump also brings about the rapid drop in Ca^{++} concentration at the end of depolarization. Most of the Ca^{++} ions present at this time in the intracellular space are rapidly taken up into the sarcoplasmic reticulum by the pump.

Figure 5-11B summarizes in diagrammatic form the manner in which muscular relaxation is initiated by the sarcoplasmic reticulum. The cell membrane is repolarized; that is to say, it once more carries a negative charge internally, and this repolarization obtains also in the transverse tubuli. Next, the membrane of the sarcoplasmic reticulum again becomes impermeable to diffusing Ca^{++} ions, and the Ca^{++} efflux is terminated. With the aid of the pump the Ca^{++} ions are again transported into the sarcoplasmic reticulum, and the contraction is brought to a stop due to the insufficient concentration of intracellular Ca^{++}.

Work through the following questions to test your knowledge of electromechanical coupling.

Q 5.9   Which of the following statements are correct? The transverse tubuli
   a. are open to the extracellular space.
   b. run transversely through the muscle fiber.
   c. are also depolarized when the outer cell membrane is depolarized.
   d. are openly connected with the sarcoplasmic reticulum.
   e. release Ca^{++} ions into the intracellular space to initiate contraction.

Q 5.10 The sarcoplasmic reticulum
   a. is open to the extracellular space.
   b. can store Ca^{++} ions.
   c. runs in the longitudinal direction of the muscle fibers.
   d. can actively take up Ca^{++} ions.
   e. regulates the intracellular K^+ concentration.

Q 5.11 Which of the following statements are correct? Contraction of the skeletal muscle fiber is triggered by
   a. depolarization of the membrane during the action potential.
   b. an increase in the intracellular Na^+ concentration during the action potential.
   c. an increase in the intracellular concentration of free Ca^{++}.
   d. an increase in the intracellular level of free ATP during membrane depolarization.
   e. inhibition of the Na^+ pump during membrane depolarization.

Q 5.12 The free Ca^{++} concentration in the relaxed muscle is, at 10^{-8} M, very low because

    a. the outer cell membrane is impermeable to Ca^{++}.

    b. a Ca^{++} pump transports Ca^{++} ions into the sarcoplasmic reticulum and thus reduces the free intracellular Ca^{++} concentration.

    c. the contractile proteins bind Ca^{++} ions to themselves and thus reduce the intracellular concentration of free Ca^{++}.

    d. Ca^{++} ions are consumed during contraction so that at the end of the contraction the free Ca^{++} concentration drops to a very low value.

5.4   Regulation of Muscular Contraction

So far in our discussion of muscular contraction we have concentrated on the individual muscle fiber and its myofibrils. However, individual fibers contract by themselves in the body very rarely, if at all; instead, contraction involves varying numbers of the fibers contained in a muscle. When a muscle contracts, many individual fibers act together, and to control the muscular force the nervous system must coordinate the activity of the individual fibers. We will now examine the way in which the contraction of the entire muscle is regulated.

Summation of the contraction of several fibers.   The contractile force of a *single muscle fiber* can be regulated, within certain limits, by the frequency with which it is excited. At very low frequencies, for example, 2/sec, the maximum force developed is that of a single contraction (twitch). If the frequency of excitation is increased, the maximum, that is, the tetanic, force can be developed by the muscle by means of summation. The tetanic force can be about five times higher than the maximum force developed in a twitch. The range in which the contractile force of a *single* fiber can be regulated by means of the frequency of excitation is thus relatively narrow.

Besides the limited summation of the contractions of the individual fibers, *summation of the twitches of parallel fibers* also takes place in the entire muscle. The parallel fibers of the muscle all end at the same tendons that combine the force they develop. This summation of the contractions of parallel fibers is illustrated by Fig. 5-12. The figure shows equal contractions of three individual fibers that are not summated because the stimulus frequencies (2 to 4/sec) are too low. The top curve in Fig. 5-12 depicts the summated contractile force of the three individual fibers at each point in time. The curve thus

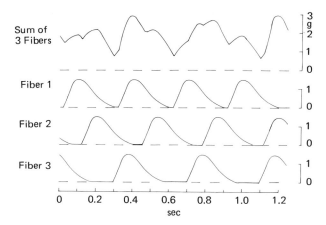

Fig. 5-12. Summation of the contraction of individual fibers. Schematic sequences of equal twitches in three parallel fibers in a muscle. The top curve is the summation curve of the contractions of the three fibers. In this curve the force never drops to zero (dotted line), whereas the contractions of the individual fibers still do not exhibit any summation.

corresponds to the force measured at a tendon in which all three fibers are combined. The maximum force in this summation curve is more than twice as high as that of the twitches, and at no point does the force drop to zero (dotted line). If the contractions of a large number of fibers were summated, the summated curve would run more uniformly and attain a higher maximum force than the summated curve in Fig. 5-12.

Muscle tonus. Summation of the twitches of many fibers, which are excited asynchronously at low frequencies up to 5/sec, generates a total force that does not fluctuate very much and whose amplitude must be approximately proportional to the average frequency of excitation. The basic tension produced in this way by summation of the twitches of many fibers is called *tone*, or *tonus*. All the muscles in a living organism possess such tone. Even in a relaxed limb the motor nerves are activated at low frequency. The resulting tone is detectable as a *resistance to passive bending of the limb*.

The tone of the muscles is chiefly involved in their *postural function*. Even when we sit relaxed, our limbs, for example, are not rendered fully passive; instead they adopt a certain attitude. This posture is determined by the relative degree of tone in the various groups of muscles. When the posture is endangered, that is, when some sort of disturbance is anticipated (example: someone is driving a car and a potential hazard situation develops on the road ahead), the tone increases, that is, the basic tension of all the muscles is increased so that the posture adopted is better fixed and more firmly held.

The tone of the muscles also plays an important role in the *thermoregulatory processes* of the organism. As described above, during each contraction, part of the converted energy appears in the form of heat, and in the case of tonic contractions, which perform no externally evident work, the energy contained in the contractions is also finally converted into heat. Thus, by varying the muscle tone the body can greatly vary the amount of heat it produces, and this capability can be put to use in regulating body temperature at various ambient temperatures. When vigorous muscular activity occurs, a great deal of heat is released by the chemical reactions, forcing the body to give off large amounts of heat, for example, by sweating.

Generation of maximum muscular force.   If the frequency of excitatory impulses in the motor nerve fibers is increased to more than 5/sec, the force of the contraction increases through summation of the twitches in the individual fibers as well as through summation of the contractions of the individual parallel fibers. The *maximum muscular force* is developed when all the individual parallel fibers develop *tetanic tension.* This force can be attained in most muscles of warmblooded animals at frequencies of about 50/sec because the summation of the contractions of many fibers compensates for the slight fluctuations in force of the individual fibers which still occur at this frequency (see Fig. 5-8*D*). Since the nerves and the motor end plates (see page 47) still function at frequencies of several 100/sec, the motor system is easily able to attain maximum contractile force.

Motor unit, electromyogram.   The statements concerning the parallel but independently contracting individual fibers need qualification. Not all the fibers are stimulated asynchronously and independently of each other. The number of motor nerve fibers that innervate the muscle is smaller than the number of muscle fibers. Within the muscle the nerve fibers branch and innervate several muscle fibers. Thus, stimulation of a single nerve fiber in each case results in simultaneous excitation of a group of muscle fibers. The motor *nerve fiber* together with the *muscle fibers which it innervates* are referred to as a *motor unit.*

The motor units vary in size. In densely innervated muscles such as the outer muscles of the eye, they contain on the average seven muscle fibers. In muscles of the lower leg they contain on the average 1,700 muscle fibers. As a result of the combining of muscle fibers in motor units, it is slightly more difficult to grade muscular contractions because all the fibers in the motor unit contract simultaneously. Therefore in muscles that must produce very finely regulated amounts of force (for example, the eye muscles), the motor units contain only a few fibers.

The excitatory impulses of the motor units can be recorded in an *electromyogram* (EMG). The EMG is an extracellular recording of the potential of the muscle. The electrodes are either placed on the skin above the muscle or inserted into the muscle (extracellularly). Figure 5-13 illustrates the electromyogram of a human eyelid muscle. No changes in potential are visible in *A*, and the muscle is fully relaxed. In *B*, *C*, and *D* the lid is closed with increasing force. In the process, extracellularly recorded action potentials, or *impulses*, show up in the electromyogram. These impulses take the form of rapid rises in potential followed by a small drop in potential. The large impulses in Fig. 5-13*B–D* all stem from one motor unit. The first five such impulses are denoted by arrows in Fig. 5-13*B*. The frequency of excitation in this motor unit increases with increasing development of force. In *B*, 13 large impulses per second can be seen for weak contraction; this figure increases to 31/sec for strong contraction (Fig. 5-13*D*). At this frequency, during strong contraction of the muscle, this motor unit probably almost attains tetanic force.

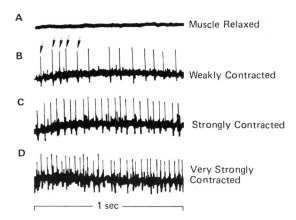

Fig. 5-13. Electromyogram of an eyelid muscle. During the recording of the electromyograms (EMGs) the muscle was fully relaxed in *A* and underwent increasing contraction in *B* to *C*. The large impulses in *B* to *D* (denoted by arrows at beginning of *B*) are all generated by one motor unit. The frequency of excitation in this motor unit increases from *A* to *D*. In addition, with stronger contraction an increasing number of small impulses is visible. These are generated by adjacent motor units. (From Bell, Davidson, and Scarborough, *Textbook of Physiology and Biochemistry*, Livingston, Edinburgh, 1968.)

Figure 5-13 shows that with increasing contractile force not only does the frequency of excitation in a single motor unit increase, but also more motor units are activated. An increasing number and variety of small pulses appear alongside the "large pulses" in C and D. These small pulses are generated by adjacent motor units which are further away from the measuring electrodes and therefore generate only small changes in potential at the electrodes. The increasing number of small pulses also shows that a larger number of motor units are activated during strong contractions.

The EMG is a much-used neurophysiological tool for diagnosing muscular diseases. These diseases take the form of paralysis or reduced ability to generate force, myasthenia, or manifest themselves in uncontrolled surplus development of force, myotonia. In many case histories the reactions of the musculature reflect damage in or disease of the motor nervous system. In other cases it is the neuromuscular transmission that is affected. Recording the excitation pattern of the motor units in the electromyogram, apart from establishing exactly the type of motor disturbance involved, is also a great aid in diagnosis. Diseases of the contractile system proper of the muscle fibers occur relatively rarely. In such cases the trouble is due to degenerative changes in the muscle fibers, muscular dystrophies, which can usually be related back to hereditary enzyme defects or hormonal disturbances.

The following questions will help you check the knowledge you have acquired in this section.

Q 5.13 Which of the following statements are correct? The contractile force of a muscle can be controlled by
    a. varying the frequency of excitation of the individual motor units.
    b. varying the number of muscle fibers that belong to a motor unit.
    c. varying the number of activated motor units.
    d. increasing the ATP level in the muscle fiber.
    e. varying the number of activated motor units *only*.

Q 5.14 Which of the following statements are correct? The electromyogram records
    a. the amplitude of muscle contraction.
    b. the duration of muscle contraction.
    c. the excitation in the motor nerve fibers.
    d. the excitation in the motor units.
    e. variations in the number of activated motor units.

Q 5.15 Which of the following statements are correct? A motor unit
    a. consists of all the muscles that together execute the same movement.

    b. consists of a motor nerve fiber with the muscle fibers that are
       innervated by it.
    c. always comprises at least 100 muscle fibers.
    d. is excited approximately simultaneously in all its elements.

6

MOTOR SYSTEMS

Those parts of the nervous system primarily responsible for the voluntary and the involuntary control of posture and movement are situated in various regions of the CNS ranging from the phylogenetically oldest part, the spinal cord, to the most recent region, the cerebral cortex. The study of the motor functions of the various brain regions revealed that the expansion of the CNS, which became necessary as the differentiation of the animal kingdom progressed, was achieved not so much by reconstructing existing regulation and control systems as by superimposing additional systems. The CNS is thus hierarchical in structure. In the following sections we shall first study the capabilities of the lowest sections in the hierarchy and then proceed to examine how far these capabilities are modified and complemented by the higher sections.

The simplest experimental way of studying the performance of the individual sections of the CNS is to remove, with appropriate transections, higher parts of the CNS. For example, if the spinal cord is separated from the rest of the CNS (spinalization) at the level of the first cervical vertebra (C_1), the motor functions of the isolated spinal cord can be studied. If the brain stem remains in contact with the spinal cord and if the sections situated higher up are eliminated (decerebration), then the influence of the brain stem on the spinal cord can be examined. Finally, removal of the cerebral cortex only (decortication) would simply lead to loss of the motor functions controlled by this particular section.

When considering the motor performance of the CNS we should bear in mind that an uninterrupted flow of afferent information is necessary to the central nervous structures involved in controlling posture and movement if they are to be able to fulfill their role. At the level of the spinal cord the dependence of motor performance on the afferent flow of information is particularly clear, because here individual types of receptors (for example, muscle spindle receptors) are connected in relatively stereotyped fashion with the motoneurons to form reflex circuits. In the first two sections of this chapter, which deal with the motor performance of the spinal cord, we shall therefore demonstrate the importance of afferent information for motor control.

6.1   Spinal Motor Systems I: Roles of Muscle Spindles and Tendon Organs

A detailed description has already been given in Sec. 4.2 of the structure of the muscle spindles and of the central connection of the Group Ia afferent fibers with the homonymous motoneurons. It was shown that the monosynaptic stretch reflex can be triggered by both stretching of the entire muscle and intrafusal contraction. It was pointed out that the first possibility is important for maintaining a given muscle length at a constant value (length servomechanism) and that the second is important for adjusting the muscle length (follow-up servomechanism). In addition, brief mention was made in Sec. 4.1 of the fact that the Group Ia fibers form not only excitatory synapses with homonymous motoneurons but also inhibitory connections with antagonistic motoneurons (see Fig. 4-4A). With this in mind, we shall now take a closer look at the central connections of the Group Ia afferent fibers and at the importance of their reflex actions for motor control, particularly for maintaining a constant muscle length. We shall then study the tendon organs (Golgi organs). These receptors are also stretch receptors. The central connections of their afferent fibers and their functions within the motor framework complement those of the muscle spindles in a manner ideally adapted to the control of posture and movement.

Stretch reflex and reciprocal antagonistic inhibition.   Figure 6-1A illustrates the segmental connections of the Ia muscle spindle afferents coming from two antagonistic muscles, taking as examples the flexor and the extensor muscles of the elbow, namely, the Musculus biceps and the M. triceps, respectively. As we have already learned in Sec. 4.2 (cf. Fig. 4-7), the Ia fibers form monosynaptic excitatory connections with their own, homonymous motoneurons. In addition, as mentioned in Sec. 4-1 (cf. Fig. 4-4A) and Sec. 4.3, collaterals of the Ia fibers form disynaptic inhibitory connections with the antagonistic motoneurons. Because it possesses the shortest inhibitory reflex arc, this is called direct inhibition. It is also termed *reciprocal* inhibition since activity in the Ia fibers results in excitation of the homonymous

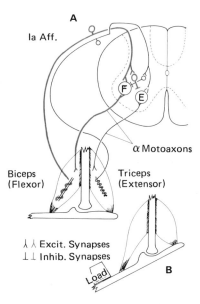

Fig. 6-1. Reflex pathways of the stretch reflex and of reciprocal antagonistic inhibition. *F*, flexor motoneuron, *E*, extensor motoneuron of the elbow joint. The flexors (biceps) and the extensors (triceps) of this joint and the polarity of the synapses are shown. The results of the passive extension of the joint by an externally acting load as shown in *B* are described in detail in the text.

motoneurons and at the same time inhibition of the antagonists. The reciprocal antagonistic inhibition thus facilitates the contraction of the homonymous (agonistic) muscle triggered by the Ia-fiber activity by simultaneously inhibiting the antagonistic muscles acting on the same joint.

It was also stated in Sec. 4.2 that the Ia fibers come from the stretch receptors of the muscle spindles and that passive stretching of the muscle (for example, in the case of the patellar reflex) leads to activation of the muscle-spindle receptors and triggers the monosynaptic stretch reflex. Using Fig. 6-1 we shall now consider the events occurring when an externally applied force changes the position of a joint. It will be seen that *all* the changes in reflex activity issuing from the muscle spindles of the *agonists* and the *antagonists* serve to reverse as far as possible the change that has occurred in the position of the joint; that is, they act to maintain the given muscle length at a *constant* value.

Let us assume that the position of the elbow joint as illustrated in Fig. 6-1*A* is disturbed by a load applied to the lower arm as shown in Fig. 6-1*B*. The stretching of the biceps will lead to increased activation of its muscle-spindle receptors, which gives rise to increased excitation of the biceps motoneurons and to increased inhibition of the triceps motoneurons. While the biceps is stretched by the load, the triceps is, at the same time, relaxed. The result of this passive shortening of the M. triceps is that the triceps muscle spindles become less activated. Consequently, the homonymous excitation of the triceps motoneurons is reduced, and the reciprocal inhibition of the biceps motoneurons is reduced (this "removal of inhibition" is also frequently termed "disinhibition").

Stretching of the elbow joint brought about by an externally applied force thus leads to increased activation of the biceps motoneurons because the homonymous excitation increases and the reciprocal antagonistic inhibition decreases. At the same time, the activity of the triceps motoneurons declines because the homonymous excitation decreases and the reciprocal antagonistic inhibition increases. Seen as a whole, the changes in activity triggered in the four mono- and disynaptic reflex arcs will tend, as far as possible, to reverse the change in the position of the joint by increasing the tension (increase in postural tone) of the biceps and reducing the tension of the triceps, that is, they will act to maintain the original muscle length at a constant value. The reflex arcs together form a *length-control system* (length servomechanism) for the muscle.

It has already been stated in Sec. 4.2 that maintenance of constant muscle length by means of the segmental reflex arcs of the Ia afferents is a typical control circuit (length servomechanism) whose various components can also be defined and simulated in the language of control technology. Apart from possessing the circuit elements that we have described so far, such a control circuit must also take account of the various time delays that occur as a result of the passage of the action potentials in the afferent and the efferent nerve fibers. In addition, it must be remembered that the discharge frequency of the muscle spindle receptors not only is proportional to the muscle length (as we have assumed for the sake of simplicity in our discussions so far) but also possesses a component that is proportional to the rate of change of the muscle length (that is, to the first derivative) (see Fig. 6-4B). To a certain extent, this second component predicts the amount by which the muscle length will change in the future, provided the change occurs at the same rate. This prediction compensates for some of the delayed reaction of the control circuit caused by the passage of the action potentials and by mass inertia.

Role of the γ loop. It has already been shown in Sec. 4.2 that it is possible to influence the output of the muscle-spindle afferents and thus to adjust the length of the muscle by efferent innervation of the intrafusal muscle fibers (γ motoaxons). We shall now take a closer look at this mechanism, but first it would perhaps be a good idea at this point to read through pages 107 to 110 of Sec. 4.2 once more.

Line a in Fig. 6-2 shows the relationship between the muscle length (abscissa) and the frequency of the Ia afferent impulses of the muscle-spindle receptors (ordinate) given a low level of γ fiber activity, that is, weak intrafusal contraction. The discharge frequency of the Ia fibers is thus directly proportional to the muscle length. Increasing the γ activity means that muscle spindles that hitherto fired at low frequency (for example, point 1 in a) now respond at a higher frequency (point 2 in b) without any change occurring in the length of the muscle. This increased activity of the Ia fibers will strongly excite the homonymous motoneurons and strongly inhibit the antagonistic motoneurons. The afferent output of the antagonistic muscle spindles is at first unchanged because, in contrast to Fig. 6-1B, the lengths of the agonist and the antagonist muscles do not change. The increased activity of the agonistic Ia fibers consequently will lead to a contraction (increase in tone) of the agonist muscle while simultaneously the antagonist is relaxed (reduction in tone), and as a result the joint in question moves. The movement will stop as soon as point 3 in line b is reached, that is, as soon as the muscle spindle afferents again transmit the same number of pulses as at point 1 of line a. The muscle length can thus be adjusted by the γ efferents *without* there being any *continuous* change in the output of the muscle-spindle receptors.

Since the change in the position of the joint stretches the antagonist muscle, the tension of the antagonistic intrafusal muscle fibers must also be changed somewhat if point 3 is to have the same

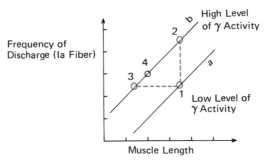

Fig. 6-2. The relationship between muscle length (abscissa) and frequency of afferent impulses from the primary endings of the muscle spindles (ordinate) for low (line a) and high (line b) activity of the γ motor nerve fibers and thus for varying tone of the intrafusal muscle fibers. The measuring points numbered 1 to 4 are explained in the text.

value on the ordinate as point 1. To bring the slightly increased afferent output from the (stretched) antagonist back to the original level, the intrafusal tension must in fact be decreased slightly. If the intrafusal tension of the antagonistic muscle spindles is not reduced, the result is increased reciprocal inhibition of the agonistic motoneurons, which, in turn, means that instead of being shortened to point 3 in Fig. 6-2, the muscle length may only reach point 4. A slightly increased agonistic Ia-impulse frequency compared with point 1 then compensates for the increased impulse frequency of the antagonistic Ia fibers.

Contraction of the musculature can be triggered either by the γ loop or by direct activation of the α motoneurons. Direct activation of the α motoneurons by supraspinal centers has the advantage that the latent period is short, but it has an apparent disadvantage in that the carefully established equilibrium of the length control system, which operates by means of the stretch reflex, is at first seriously disrupted. As a result, the affected muscle spindles may no longer be adequately stretched (subthreshold stretching), or they may be overstretched (saturation). On the other hand, activation of the γ loop causes contraction of the muscle without or with only a brief change in the spindle output. It seems reasonable to assume that predominant direct excitation of the α motoneurons is utilized above all when speed is important, while activation of the γ loop makes smooth and precise movements possible. Unfortunately, we still know very little about the relative importance of the two forms of activitation. However, recent recordings from motor nerves of man have shown that at least in voluntary movements there is usually *a coactivation of the α and the γ pathways.*

Position and discharge pattern of muscle spindles and Golgi organs.   Apart from the muscle-spindle receptors, the skeletal muscles contain another type of stretch receptor that is important for motor control. This is the *Golgi organ*, also called the tendon organ. The position of the Golgi organs in the muscle differs from that of the muscle spindles, resulting in different discharge patterns for the two types of receptor, particularly during contraction. Figure 6-3 illustrates the position of two Golgi organs and one muscle-spindle receptor (only one intrafusal muscle fiber is shown) in the muscle. The afferent nerve terminal of the muscle–spindle receptor winds itself around the central part of the intrafusal muscle fiber, while the Golgi organs are located at the *tendons* of the extrafusal muscle fibers. The figure shows further that the Golgi organ afferents are called Ib fibers. As in the case of the Ia fibers of the muscle spindles, the Ib fibers of

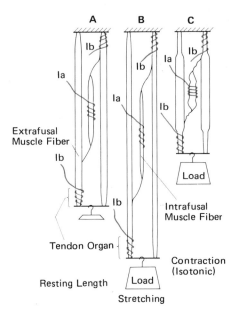

Fig. 6-3. Sketch showing the position of the muscle spindles and the tendon organs in the muscle and illustrating their changes in shape during stretching (*B*) and isotonic contraction (*C*).

the tendon organs are thick, myelinated fibers whose conduction velocity is as high as that of the Ia fibers, approximately 75 m/sec (see Table 2-2).

If the muscle is stretched (*B* in Fig. 6-3) from the resting length (*A*), then both the muscle spindles and the tendon organs are stretched. During subsequent isotonic contraction (*C*) the tendon organs continue to remain stretched while the load on the muscle spindles is removed. These results are frequently expressed in the following way: the muscle spindle is connected *in parallel* and the tendon organ *in series* with the extrafusal musculature. Because of this dissimilarity, the discharge patterns of the muscle spindles and the tendon organs are characteristically different during contraction of the extrafusal muscle fibers.

Figure 6-4 shows discharge patterns of muscle spindle (Ia) afferents and tendon organ (Ib) afferents at rest (*A*), when stretched (*B*), and during contraction (*C*). The threshold of the tendon organs for passive stretching is somewhat higher than that of the muscle spindles, so that for a given muscle length (cf. Ia with Ib in *A* and in the final one-third of *B*) the discharge frequency of the muscle spindles is higher than that of the tendon organs. During stretch (*B*) the discharge frequency of both the Ia and the Ib fibers increases. While the stretch-

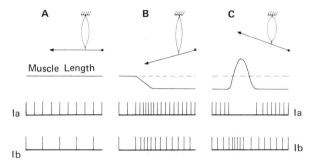

Fig. 6-4. Discharge patterns of muscle spindles (by Ia fibers) and of tendon organs (by Ib fibers) at rest (A), stretched (B), and during isotonic contraction (C).

ing occurs, the discharge frequency is higher than when the new length is reached. This indicates that the discharge frequency of both stretch receptors is proportional not only to the length of the muscle but also to the rate at which the length changes (that is, it is proportional to the first derivative of the change in length with time). This component is much more pronounced in the case of muscle spindles than of tendon organs.

Contraction of the extrafusal muscle fibers (C in Fig. 6-4) removes the load from the muscle spindles and thus terminates the Ia discharges. The tendon organ remains stretched (see also Fig. 6-3C), and its discharge frequency increases temporarily during the isotonic contraction because the acceleration of the load leads to a brief but strong stretching of the tendon organ. It can be concluded that the *muscle spindles* primarily measure the *length* of the muscle, while the *tendon organs* primarily record the *tension*. It is to be expected therefore that during isometric contraction (that is, when tension is increased without a change in length) the discharge frequency of the tendon organs will increase strongly, while that of the muscle spindles should remain approximately constant [de facto the discharge rate of the muscle spindles actually decreases because, despite the constant external length, the contractile elements inside the muscle undergo shortening at the expense of the elastic elements (see also Sec. 5.2) with the result that load is removed from the muscle spindles].

Segmental connections of the Ib fibers and roles of the Golgi organs. In functional terms the segmental connections of the Ib fibers (Fig. 6-5) mirror those of the Ia fibers (cf. Fig. 6-1A). The tendon organs form *inhibitory* connections with their *homonymous* motoneurons and *excitatory* connections with *antagonistic* motoneurons. However, there are no monosynaptic connections with the motoneu-

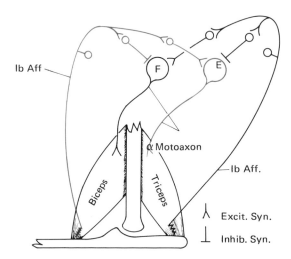

Fig. 6-5. Segmental connections of Ib fibers from the tendon organs in the muscle. Diagram similar to Fig. 6-1.

rons. Both the excitatory and the inhibitory connections are at least disynaptic; that is, they are just as long as the reflex arc of reciprocal antagonistic inhibition mediated by the Ia fibers. Since the tendon organs measure the *tension* of the muscle, a strong increase in muscle tension—whether caused by passive stretch, active contraction, or a combination of the two—will lead to inhibition of the homonymous motoneurons via the Ib fibers and thus prevent too strong a rise in tension (with the attendant danger of the muscle or tendon tearing). As can be demonstrated clearly in decerebrate animals, increased stretch of a muscle leads to increasing muscle tension (by the stretch reflex arc) until, when the stretch is severe, the muscle tone suddenly declines. This phenomenon is called the *clasp-knife reflex* and is ascribed to the inhibitory effect of the homonymous tendon organs. It has been concluded from this that the role of the Ib reflex arc is mainly that of a *protective reflex*.

However, the role of the tendon organs as protection against over-stretching of the muscle is probably only one aspect of the tendon organ's function. In fact, while an increase in muscle tension leads by the tendon organs to inhibition of the homonymous motoneurons, a decrease in muscle tension will lead to a drop in the impulse activity in the Ib fibers, causing disinhibition (removal of inhibition) of the homonymous motoneurons; as a result the muscle tension should increase again. In other words, the reflex arc of the tendon organs is connected in such a way that it can serve to keep the *tension* of the muscle *constant*. Each muscle thus possesses two feedback systems (control circuits): a length control system, with the muscle spindles as sensors, and a tension control system, with the tendon organs as sensors.

Technically speaking it is not immediately apparent why it is necessary to have both a tension control system and a length control system. In an ideal length control circuit the force developed by the muscle would always be proportional to the efferent pulses in the α motoaxons, and a tension control system would be superfluous. But, as we know from Chapter 5, the force developed by the muscle is also dependent on the amount of prestretching, the rate of contraction, and the degree of fatigue of the muscle. The deviations of the muscle tension from the desired value, as a result of these factors, are measured by the tendon organs and corrected by the tension control system.

Please answer the following questions to check the new knowledge you have acquired.

Q 6.1 Which of the following statements is/are correct?
   a. The muscle spindles are connected in parallel with the intrafusal musculature.
   b. The tendon organs are connected in series with the extrafusal musculature.
   c. The tendon organs are innervated by Ia afferents.
   d. The Ib afferents form disynaptic excitatory connections with homonymous motoneurons.
   e. The efferent innervation of the tendon organs is achieved via γ fibers.
   f. All the above statements are false.

Q 6.2 Which of the following inputs to a motoneuron have an excitatory effect?
   a. Afferent activity from homonymous muscle spindles.
   b. Afferent activity from homonymous tendon organs.
   c. Afferent activity from antagonistic muscle spindles.
   d. Afferent activity from antagonistic tendon organs.

Q 6.3 Increased activity of the γ efferents of a flexor muscle
   a. does not change the position of the joint.
   b. causes extension of the joint via the tension control system.
   c. increases the tone of the flexor and the extensor muscles while leaving the position of the joint unchanged.
   d. results in reflex flexing of the joint.
   e. reduces the Ia activity of the antagonistic extensor.

Q 6.4 The clasp-knife reflex (sudden easing of muscle tone during extreme stretching) is caused by
   a. strong excitation of the homonymous muscle spindles.
   b. strong excitation of the antagonistic muscle spindles.

    c. complete removal of the load from the antagonistic muscle spindles.

    d. strong excitation of the homonymous tendon organs.

    e. complete removal of the load from the heteronymous tendon organs.

Q 6.5 Which receptor type is the sensor in the
    a. length control system of the muscle.
    b. tension control system of the muscle.

6.2   Spinal Motor Systems II: Polysynaptic Motor Reflexes; the Flexor Reflex

In the preceding section we discussed the roles of the receptors located in the muscle itself, the muscle spindles and the tendon organs. Many of the other receptors of the body, for example, those of the skin, can also trigger motor reflexes (see examples in Sec. 4.3). Experiments on spinal animals have shown that for many of these the reflex arcs run in the spinal cord. Common to all is the fact that they are polysynaptic; that is, more than one interneuron is located along their reflex pathway in the spinal cord. In the following we shall learn about the most important of these polysynaptic spinal motor reflexes and their characteristics. The most prominent example is the *flexor reflex* which we shall therefore make the starting point and the central subject of our remarks. However, we shall see that other reflex arcs are always activated with the flexor reflex. The main role of these other reflexes is to ensure that the disruptions of the body's balance caused by the flexor reflex are checked and compensated. In the last part of this section we shall see what reflex activity the isolated human spinal cord is capable of performing. This is of great practical importance since transections of the spinal cord in man are becoming more and more frequent as a result of accidents, particularly traffic accidents. The clinical picture is referred to as paraplegia.

Flexor reflex and crossed extensor reflex.   If a painful stimulus is applied to a hind paw of a spinal animal (pinching, strong electric shock, heat) then the animal withdraws the stimulated extremity; that is, flexion occurs in the ankle joint, the knee joint, and the hip joint. This phenomenon is referred to as the *flexor reflex*. Painful stimulation of a front paw likewise causes withdrawal of the affected extremity, again a flexor reflex. In this case the ankle joint, the elbow joint, and the shoulder joint are flexed. The receptors (nociceptors) of this reflex are located in the skin of the limbs, and the effectors are the flexor muscles. It is therefore an *extrinsic reflex*. Obviously the role of the flexor reflex is to remove the limb from the site where it is exposed to painful stimulation. It is thus a typical *protective reflex*. If we press the paw of an animal with varying degrees of force it will be found that the reaction time and the size of the reflex response depend to a large extent on the intensity of the stimulus. As the intensity of the stimulus increases, the reaction time becomes shorter, and the withdrawal of the limb occurs more briskly. This possibility of summation, as we have seen in Sec. 4.3, is a typical characteristic of *polysynaptic* reflexes. We can conclude that the flexor reflex, seen in terms of the anatomical position of the receptors and the effectors, is an extrinsic reflex. Its appearance in spinal animals and its characteristics show that it possesses a spinal polysynaptic reflex arc. In functional terms it is a protective reflex.

When palpating the musculature of a limb during a flexor reflex it can be felt that the *extensors* relax during flexion. This indicates that during this reflex the extensor motoneurons of the flexed limb are inhibited. It can be observed further that the flexion of a hind or a fore limb is always accompanied by extension of the opposite (contralateral) limb. Painful stimulation of an extremity thus results ipsilaterally in a flexor reflex and contralaterally in an *extensor reflex*. The contralateral extensor reflex is also called a *crossed extensor reflex* because the afferent activity coming from the nociceptors crosses to the other (contralateral) side of the spinal cord where it induces the extensor reflex. If we palpate the contralateral limb during the crossed extensor reflex we find that the flexor muscles relax during the extension of the limb. This indicates that during excitation of the contralateral extensor motoneurons, the contralateral flexor motoneurons are inhibited.

It is obvious that altogether four motor reflex arcs are activated at the segmental level as a result of painful stimulation of a limb: (1) an excitation of all ipsilateral flexor motoneurons (all the joints are flexed = flexor reflex), (2) an inhibition of the ipsilateral extensor motoneurons, (3) an excitation of the contralateral extensor motoneurons (crossed extensor reflex), and (4) an inhibition of the contralateral flexor motoneurons. Experimental electrophysiological analysis of the flexor reflex and its accompanying reflexes has confirmed the hypotheses advanced so far regarding the pathways of these reflexes. Figure 6-6 shows diagrammatically the segmental polysynaptic pathways activated by an afferent fiber arising from a cutaneous nociceptor. The ipsilateral flexor motoneurons are excited, and the ipsilateral extensor motoneurons are inhibited through several interneurons (only two are shown in each case). In addition, the ipsilateral afferent activity from

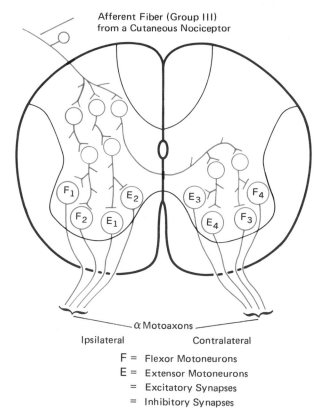

Afferent Fiber (Group III)
from a Cutaneous Nociceptor

Ipsilateral   Contralateral

α Motoaxons

F = Flexor Motoneurons
E = Extensor Motoneurons
   = Excitatory Synapses
   = Inhibitory Synapses

Fig. 6-6. Intrasegmental connections of an afferent fiber arising from a cutaneous nociceptor. The function of the motoneurons and the polarity of the synapses are discussed in the text.

the nociceptors is transmitted to the contralateral side by interneurons whose axons cross in the anterior commissure. Here, likewise, via polysynaptic reflex arcs, the extensor motoneurons are excited and the flexor motoneurons are inhibited.

Not everyone has the opportunity to study the flexor reflex, the crossed extensor reflex, and the associated reciprocal inhibitions on the spinal animal in the laboratory. However, the flexor reflex can easily be observed without spinalization in newborn domestic animals or those which are just a few days old or in human infants, because at this very early age the higher regions of the brain are not fully matured, and therefore the simple spinal reflex patterns are not yet obscured by more complicated patterns.

Intersegmental reflex pathways.   If all the dorsal roots of a spinal cord are transected and if, in addition, the cord is separated from the higher (rostral or cranial) sections of the brain, then all the fibers in this "isolated spinal cord" whose cells are not located in the spinal cord degenerate (die). That is, all the dorsal root fibers—cells located in the dorsal root (spinal) ganglia—and all the (descending) axons entering the spinal cord from the cranial region die. In such specimens the gray matter remains practically unchanged since it contains the somata of the neurons of the spinal cord. Surprisingly, however, the surrounding white matter, which is formed by the ascending and the descending axons, is also only slightly reduced. This permits us to conclude that most axons that come from the neurons of the gray matter end inside the spinal cord. Neurons whose axons project and terminate within the spinal cord are called *propriospinal neurons.* Ascending or descending bundles of axons (nerve fibers) originating and terminating within the spinal cord are called *propriospinal pathways.*

Most neurons of the gray matter of the spinal cord are therefore propriospinal neurons. This anatomical finding alone indicates the great importance of the connections between the individual segments of the spinal cord. Figure 6-7 shows that an afferent fiber, along with

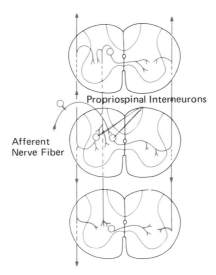

Fig. 6-7.   Intersegmental connections of an afferent nerve fiber. After it enters the spinal cord the afferent fiber branches into segmental, ascending, and descending collaterals that terminate on interneurons. The axons of these interneurons either terminate within the spinal cord (propriospinal neurons) or lead to supraspinal structures.

its segmental (Figs. 6-1, 6-5, 6-6) and supraspinal (see Sec. 7.2) connections, usually possesses several pathways to neighboring and more
distant segments. First, an afferent fiber splits up into several collaterals after it enters the spinal cord, and some of these collaterals link up
directly with neighboring segments without any relaying via an interneuron. In addition, collaterals of the afferent fibers form excitatory
synapses with propriospinal interneurons at the level of the entry
zone; the axons of these interneurons form either ipsilateral or, after
crossing in the anterior commissure, contralateral reflex connections.

Details of the propriospinal pathways will not be dealt with here.
At this point, it is sufficient to know that in some pathways the
propriospinal axons are very short (a few millimeters or even less,
projecting only into their immediate surroundings), while others, as
indicated in Fig. 6-7, extend over many segments. The *role of the
propriospinal pathways* is to connect the individual spinal segments
with one another. Thus they form *intersegmental* reflex arcs. For
example, in the case of a spinal animal, painful stimulation of a limb
gives rise not only to a crossed extensor reflex but also to an excitation
of the extensor motoneurons of the two other extremities. If the painful stimulus is long-lasting this extension can turn into a rhythmic
stretching and flexing of all three nonstimulated limbs; that is, it can
give rise to a running action.

Reflex functions of the isolated spinal cord.   Standing and running reflexes can also be triggered in the spinal animal by nonpainful
stimulation, such as pressure on the soles of the feet (see also Sec. 6.1).
All these experiments stress the fact that the interconnections of the
neurons of the spinal cord permit complex motor movements to be
carried out and coordinated when a suitable input is received from the
periphery or from the higher sections of the CNS. We call this the
integrative function of the spinal cord. However, we are far from fully
understanding the functional significance of all the spinal reflex arcs
known to us. The Renshaw inhibition in Fig. 4-4 is an example of this.
This pathway leads from motoaxon collaterals (which branch off from
the motoaxons within the spinal cord) via an inhibitory interneuron
(Renshaw cell) back to the motoneurons. It is a negative feedback
circuit of a type frequently encountered in the CNS and in electrical
engineering, and as such its role is certainly to prevent uncontrolled
oscillation of motoneuronal activity. However, its exact significance in
the spinal cord is still unknown.

In the higher vertebrates, particularly in mammals, the higher
regions of the CNS have increasingly assumed control of the spinal
cord functions; consequently, the isolated spinal cord is capable to

only a very modest extent of carrying out control and regulatory functions. In man, transection of the spinal cord results in immediate and permanent paralysis of all voluntary movements of the muscles which are served by spinal cord segments located caudally from the injury site (*paraplegia*). Conscious sensations from the affected dermatomes are likewise permanently lost. All reflexes are also, to start with, extinguished (areflexia). Some of them are later recovered to a limited extent, and some of them become even stronger than before. The muscles are at first flaccid, and reflexes (for example, stretch reflexes during passive movement) cannot be elicited. Provided the patient receives correct care, a flexor reflex appears after about two weeks when the sole of the foot is vigorously rubbed. In this case the toes are stretched toward the dorsum of the foot and spread apart (this is known as Babinski's reflex). After a month the flexor reflexes can become extraordinarily strong, and their occurrence is often accompanied by strong, vegetative reflexes, such as outbreaks of sweating, bladder contraction, and rectal contraction. Extensor reflexes develop more slowly than the flexor reflexes and are usually not very pronounced. All the vegetative (autonomic) reflexes (see Sec. 8.4) also disappear fully at first and return, to varying degrees, only after several months have elapsed. Deviations from this clinical picture, above all strong extensor reflexes and increased muscle tone shortly after the injury, are usually a sign of incomplete transection of the spinal cord with correspondingly better prospects of improvement in motor function and sensation.

The reversible neurological deficits that are manifest after spinal transection are referred to collectively as *spinal shock*. It can be shown in animal experiments that even a functional transection caused by local cooling or local anesthesia can provoke spinal shock. After an initial transection and recovery of the reflexes a second transection below the first site will no longer elicit a spinal shock. Obviously, the decisive factor governing the latter is the breakdown of the connection with the remainder of the CNS. We possess only very incomplete and unsatifactory knowledge of the causes of spinal shock and the mechanisms which bring about recovery of the reflexes. If one assumes that, as a result of transection of the descending pathways, a large number of excitatory effects acting on α or γ motoneurons and on other spinal neurons are lost, and that perhaps, in addition, inhibitory spinal interneurons become disinhibited so that altogether there is a strong suppression of reflexes, then the question arises immediately as to what mechanisms are responsible for the return of some spinal cord functions and why the recovery period takes many months. A number of individual observations have given rise to various hypotheses regarding these processes. However, experimental confirmation or refutation of these proposed hypotheses is still largely a matter for future research.

Please work through the following questions to check your knowledge of polysynaptic motor reflexes.

Q 6.6   Which of the following terms fit the flexor reflex? (Choose three!)
a. Intrinsic reflex.
b. Extrinsic reflex.
c. Monosynaptic reflex.
d. Disynaptic reflex.
e. Polysynaptic reflex.
f. Nutritional reflex.
g. Protective reflex.
h. Locomotive reflex.

Q 6.7   Which spinal afferent can activate the flexor reflex?
a. Ia fibers of the primary muscle spindle receptors.
b. Group III fibers from the nociceptors of the skin.
c. Ib fibers of the Golgi tendon organ receptors.
d. Each spinal afferent can activate the flexor reflex given very strong suprathreshold stimulation.

Q 6.8   Painful stimulation of a limb activates the flexor reflex arc. Accompanying this, one observes
a. inhibition of the ipsilateral flexor motoneurons.
b. inhibition of the ipsilateral extensor motoneurons.
c. excitation of the contralateral flexor motoneurons.
d. excitation of the contralateral extensor motoneurons.
e. inhibition of the contralateral flexor motoneurons.

Q 6.9   If, in animal experiments, the spinal cord is fully isolated from both afferent and descending connections, then all the axons whose cells are not situated in the spinal cord degenerate. The white matter than contains only propriospinal pathways and it
a. disappears completely.
b. is reduced to less than half of its original extent.
c. is only slightly reduced.
d. is fully retained.
e. is fully retained, but the gray matter disappears.

Q 6.10 Transection of the spinal cord in man leads to spinal shock. During spinal shock
a. all motor reflexes and autonomic reflexes are extinguished.
b. the motor reflexes are extinguished, but the autonomic reflexes are boosted.
c. the extensor reflexes are extinguished, but the flexor reflexes are boosted.
d. all reflexes remain unchanged.

6.3 The Functional Anatomy of Supramedullary Motor Centers

The CNS is usually divided into individual regions according to phylogenetic age. Within these regions accumulations of anatomically and functionally related neurons are differentiated from each other as *nuclei* or *ganglia*. The bundles of nerve fibers (axons) that link the individual sections of the brain with each other are called *tracts*, or *pathways*. The tracts appear white in undyed histological sections because of the medullated sheaths of the myelinated fibers, while the nuclear regions appear gray (buy a brain from the butcher and cut it longitudinally and transversely). In the spinal cord the gray matter, that is, the somata of the neurons, is surrounded by white matter (see Fig. 1-11). In the cerebrum the reverse is the case: the cerebral cortex appears gray, because it contains the somata of the cortical cells, while the axons leading to the brain stem make the underlying tissue appear white.

The exact course of the individual pathways in the brain can be established experimentally by transection studies since nerve fibers (axons) always die (degenerate) within a few days after separation from their soma. For example, degeneration of a nerve fiber bundle below (in a caudal direction from) the site of transection means that the cell bodies of these axons are situated above (in cranial direction from) the site of transection. The axons in question must therefore be part of an efferent pathway leading from the center to the periphery. By means of this technique it has been possible to show many, but by no means all, of the longitudinal and the transverse connections of the CNS. Electrophysiological stimulation and recording techniques nowadays supplement the histological methods.

In this section we shall give a brief and very simplified description of the most important nuclear regions in the motor system and of their pathways, without attempting a phylogenetic classification. In this description a large number of small nuclear areas have been grouped together into functionally larger units (centers), particularly in the brain stem. We will not go into the histology of the individual nuclear regions. The fine structure of the cerebral cortex will be mentioned and that of the cerebellar cortex will be outlined. The latter is a relatively simple structure, and we know enough about the links between the individual cells to permit us to draw certain conclusions about their function (see Sec. 6.5). It must be stressed that the anatomy of the supramedullary central nervous structures is a difficult subject regarding both the macroscopic and the fine structure of the individual sections. For the student who wishes to go into this in more detail, there are a number of textbooks that can be consulted.

Supraspinal motor centers; nomenclature, position in the CNS.
The spinal cord contains the motoneurons, and, as we have seen, it is
capable of many complex motor functions. Cranial to the spinal cord
(supraspinal), however, there are other important motor centers whose
functions we must know. A total of four supraspinal motor centers are
shown in the block diagram of Fig. 6-8. These four centers are called
the *brain stem*, the *basal ganglia*, the *motor cortex*, and the
cerebellum. It will be noticed that the brain stem, the basal ganglia,
and the motor cortex are connected *in series*, while the cerebellum is
connected *in parallel* with the other motor centers. All the efferent
motor pathways are drawn in red, and the afferent pathways are
shown in black. The shaded arrows indicate the connections between
the cerebral cortex and the cerebellar cortex (cerebrocerebellar
tracts).

In the efferent pathways, the most important synaptic relays are
indicated by the breaks in the pathways. It will be noticed that one of
the two pathways leads without interruption from the motor cortex to
the spinal cord, while the other pathway is interrupted twice, in the
basal ganglia and the brain stem. The pathway which leads without
interruption from the motor cortex to the spinal cord is called the
corticospinal pathway or *Tractus corticospinalis*. The corticospinal
pathway passes through a structure in the brain stem called the

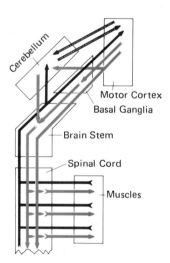

Fig. 6-8. Block diagram of spinal and supraspinal motor centers and their
most important connections. Afferent (centripetal) pathways are indicated in
black, efferent (centrifugal) pathways in red. The connections between the
cerebral cortex (motor cortex) and the cerebellum (cerebrocerebellar pathways) are indicated by the shaded arrows.

pyramid. Therefore the corticospinal pathway is also known as the *pyramidal tract.* All the other efferent motor pathways that do not pass through the pyramid are taken together as *extrapyramidal* pathways. There are a large number of extrapyramidal pathways, particularly from the brain stem to the spinal cord. Their names are usually derived from the origin and the destination of their neurons (for example, Tractus reticulospinalis, vestibulospinalis, rubrospinalis, and so on).

The red-shaded areas in Fig. 6-9 show the approximate position of

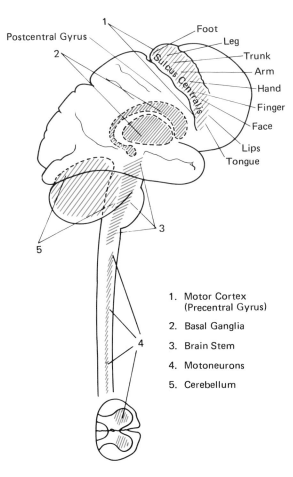

Fig. 6-9. Anatomical position of spinal and supraspinal motor centers (red shading). The motor centers are numbered 1 to 5, and their nomenclature is given to the right of the illustration. The figure also shows the somatotopic organization of the Gyrus praecentralis.

the motor centers of the brain and the spinal cord as seen from a lateral viewpoint. All the motor centers are arranged in pairs, that is, they each occur once in the right- and left-hand halves of the brain as indicated in the diagrammatic cross section through the spinal cord which is given for the motoneuron nuclei at the bottom of Fig. 6-9. The motor centers of the brain stem include a series of small nuclear regions that are distributed over the entire brain stem. Therefore the red shading in that section is to be taken only as an approximate guide. The basal ganglia, on the other hand, are very clearly delineated large nuclear structures of which the most important are the *striatum* (putamen and caudatum) and the *pallidum*. The basal ganglia are located in the immediate vicinity of the thalamus, which is the most important sensory nuclear region of the brain. All these nuclei are covered by the cerebral cortex; therefore they are not visible from outside and can be reached only through the cerebral cortex. On the other hand, the *motor cortex* is situated to a large extent at the surface of the cerebral cortex. The most important, but not the only, cortical motor area is the Gyrus praecentralis, located in front of the central sulcus (Sulcus centralis). The pyramidal tract (Tractus corticospinalis) starts from here as well as from surrounding areas.

The *cerebellum* is clearly demarcated from the rest of the brain but is connected with it by thick peduncles forming afferent and efferent pathways (see arrows in Fig. 6-8). The cerebellum receives exact "carbon copies" of the afferent and the efferent flow of information from and to the motor centers by axon collaterals and special pathways (arrows leading *to* the cerebellum). Messages can be transmitted from the cerebellum to the cerebral cortex (shaded arrow leading *from* the cerebellum), or also (red arrow leading *from* the cerebellum) directly to the motor centers in the brain stem by way of the extrapyramidal pathways. The clear differences in appearance between the cerebral and the cerebellar cortex are caused by the different arrangement of the neurons and their axons in these cortical regions. Therefore, even an inexperienced person can recognize the cerebellum in a preparation of the brain. Like the cerebrum, the cerebellar cortex encloses several nuclear regions. These cerebellar nuclei are relays for the impulses leaving the cerebellar cortex.

The pyramidal tract. Figure 6-10 shows the course of the Tractus corticospinalis, the pyramidal tract, in more detail. The cells of origin are located in the *motor cortex*, that is, in and around the Gyrus praecentralis. The axons of the pyramidal pathway run without interruption into the spinal cord. This means that in man some of these axons must be over 1 m long. The axons of the pyramidal tract run at

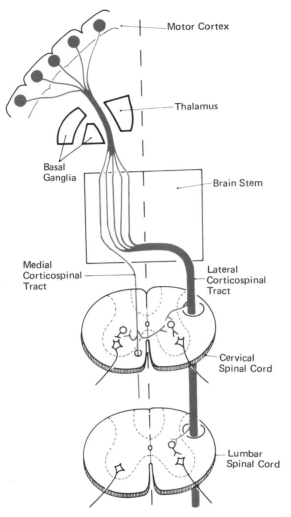

Fig. 6-10. Diagram of the course of the pyramidal tract (red) from the motor cortex to the spinal cord. See text for details.

first between the thalamus and the basal ganglia into the brain stem. This region is called the *Capsula interna* (internal capsule) of the brain, because here the pyramidal tract and other pathways surround the thalamus like a capsule. This region is very important clinically because it is here that hemorrhage or thrombosis of the blood vessels (for example, as a result of arteriosclerosis) frequently cause a block of impulse conduction with potentially fatal effects (this is known as a stroke or apoplexy).

From the Capsula interna the pyramidal tract enters the *brain stem*. The greater part of the fibers cross the midline to the other side and, after crossing, run caudally (downward) in the posterolateral quadrant of the spinal cord. The remaining fibers run uncrossed in a caudal direction in the anteromedial sections of the spinal cord. This section of the pyramidal tract usually reaches the cervical and the thoracic regions of the spinal cord but not the lumbar region. Of the approximately 1,000,000 fibers contained in each corticospinal tract (only one tract is drawn in Fig. 6-10) 75 to 90 percent cross in the lower section of the brain stem (because of its shape the area of crossing is called the *pyramid*). The other axons remain ipsilateral. Interruption of a pyramidal tract in the internal capsule thus will lead chiefly to clinical symptoms on the side contralateral to the lesion.

The axons of the pyramidal tract end in the *spinal cord*. Some of the uncrossed axons cross at the segmental level to the contralateral side so that the percentage of crossed axons is still further increased. Only a few of the pyramidal tract axons end directly on motoneurons. For the most part, they act on the motoneurons through segmental interneurons. The axons projecting from a circumscribed area of the motor cortex always act on particular peripheral muscles; that is, the *motor cortex* is *somatotopically* organized. This somatotopic organization is shown in Fig. 6-9 for the Gyrus praecentralis. The pyramidal cells related to the foot are situated most medially. Those of the face, the lips, and the tongue are situated most laterally. It will be noted that the areas of the fore limb and of the face take up a particularly large amount of space in the Gyrus praecentralis. The functional significance of this finding will be explained in Sec. 6.5.

In summary, the corticospinal tracts originate in cells of the motor cortex. The majority of the corticospinal axons cross in the brain stem to the contralateral side and run in a caudal direction in the lateral corticospinal tract of the spinal cord. At the segmental level the axons of the pyramidal tract end primarily on interneurons. Certain groups of muscles are associated with particular areas of the motor cortex. The motor cortex is thus said to be somatotopically organized.

Extrapyramidal pathways. All other efferent motor pathways originating from the motor cortex and other supraspinal centers differ in two ways from the pyramidal tracts. First, axons of these pathways do not cross in the pyramid; therefore they are called *extrapyramidal* pathways. Second, as Figs. 6-8 and 6-11 show, all the extrapyramidal pathways have one or more synapses along their route to the spinal cord. For example, all extrapyramidal pathways issuing from the motor cortex project no further than the brain stem and often end sooner in the basal ganglia of the cerebrum, for example, in the striatum or the pallidum.

Figure 6-11 shows the four most important extrapyramidal path-

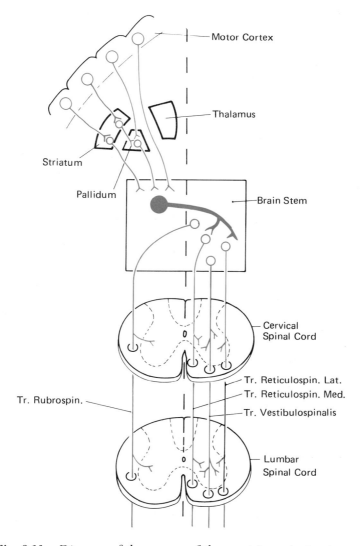

Fig. 6-11. Diagram of the course of the most important extrapyramidal pathways (red) from the supraspinal motor centers to the spinal cord. The thickly drawn neuron in the brain stem symbolizes that most extrapyramidal motor pathways cross to the contralateral side in the brain stem. The connections of the brain stem structures involved in the motor system are extremely complex in detail and are shown here in only simplified form.

ways between motor cortex and brain stem: (1) directly from the
cortex to the brain stem (through the Capsula interna); (2) and (3) a
single synaptic relay either in the striatum or in the pallidum; (4) two
synaptic relays, the first one in the striatum and the second one in the
pallidum (not the other way around). These axons end in the brain
stem without crossing to the other side. A series of extrapyramidal
motor pathways, then, originates in the brain stem. Four such pathways are shown in Fig. 6-11. Their names are derived from their site
of origin in the brain stem (Formatio reticularis, vestibular nuclei,
Nucleus ruber) and from their course in the spinal cord (med., lat.).
They are called Tractus reticulospinalis lateralis, Tractus reticulospinalis medialis, Tractus vestibulospinalis, Tractus rubrospinalis.

Because of the complex intermeshing of the pathways entering the
brain stem, not all of which arrive from the motor cortex (see Fig. 6-8,
where efferents from the cerebellum are also shown), it is not possible
to relate individual extrapyramidal pathways from the motor cortex
directly to a given tract descending to the spinal cord. Figure 6-11
shows, however, that the activity originating in the motor cortex is
transmitted, for the most part, by neurons of the brain stem to the
reticulospinal pathways of the other side. The axons of the reticulospinal pathways run uncrossed, so that, seen from the peripheral
muscle, the influences of the contralateral motor cortex predominate
in the extrapyramidal pathways as well. The Tractus rubrospinalis and
vestibulospinalis are examples of extrapyramidal pathways whose inputs, for the most part, do *not* arise from the motor cortex. The most
important influences here are those of the cerebellum (Tractus rubrospinalis) and of the vestibular organ (Tractus vestibulospinalis). It
must be remembered that the extrapyramidal motor pathways, in
contrast to the pyramidal tract, originate not only in the motor cortex
but also in other brain structures, such as the cerebellum and the
vestibular nuclei (nuclear regions of the vestibular organ). With the
exception of the basal ganglia, all the important supraspinal relays of
the extrapyramidal motor pathways are located in the brain stem.

We are now familiar with the anatomical location of the most
important motor centers of the nervous system and their main inter-
connecting pathways. We will, by and large, ignore their microscopic
structure—the arrangement and the connection of the neurons occurring in the individual nuclear regions—because at the present time
too little is known about the relationships between the function of the
supraspinal regions of the brain and their microstructure. In this
regard the best understood component is the cerebellar cortex whose
relatively simple histological structure (see page 170, structure of the
cerebellar cortex) facilitates research into the physiological function

of this part of the brain. On the other hand, the motor cortex, like the entire cerebral cortex, is much more complex in structure and thus much more difficult to analyze. Therefore we will touch only briefly upon its structure.

Structure of the motor cortex.   In the motor cortex, as in the entire cerebral cortex, layers composed predominantly of cell bodies alternate with layers containing mainly axons so that the freshly sectioned cortex presents a striated appearance. Typically, on the basis of the cell shapes and their arrangement, six different layers are identifiable, of which several are further divided into two or more sublayers. The total thickness of these six layers varies between 1.5 and 4.5 mm in the human cortex, whose surface area is approximately 2,200 cm². Also, the appearance and the relative thickness of the individual layers vary in different parts of the cortex. Systematic microscopic study of these differences has led to the compilation of brain charts in which the various cerebral regions of identical histological structure are entered. On the basis of physiological tests and clinical findings, these histological regions may be associated to some extent with those areas to which certain functions are ascribed. For example, the Gyrus postcentralis (mainly sensory functions) can be easily distinguished on the basis of fine structure from the Gyrus praecentralis, which possesses mainly motor functions.

The Gyrus praecentralis is characterized above all by its considerable thickness of 3.5 to 4.5 mm and by the *giant pyramidal cells* (Betz cells, diameter 50 to 100 μ) in the fifth cortical layer (numbered from the surface). These and smaller pyramidal cells in the third layer are the cells of origin of the pyramidal tract. Their axons run downward in the direction of the internal capsule. The majority of their dendrites run toward the surface of the cortex. The pyramidal cells were named because of the particular shape of their somata long before it was known that they are the cells of origin of the pyramidal tract. This similarity of names is thus purely accidental. There are pyramidal cells in other areas of the brain as well. The fastest axons of the pyramidal tract (conduction velocity 60 to 90 m/sec) issue from these giant pyramidal cells, but they account for only about 3 percent (30,000 out of 10^6 per each half of the brain) of the pyramidal axons. All the remainder conduct much more slowly. Pyramidal tract neurons, whose axons carry the integrated information from the cerebral cortex to the periphery, are much less numerous than the cortical neurons whose axons remain within the cortex or run to other ipsilateral or contralateral sections of the brain. The latter serve to process the cortical information and are referred to as *association neurons*, whereas the former are called *projection neurons*. On the whole the association neurons are situated more in the surface cortical layers while the projection neurons occur at deeper levels.

Structure of the cerebellar cortex.   In contrast to the cerebral cortex the *cerebellar cortex* has only three clearly distinct layers, which are practically the same in appearance in all regions of the cerebellar cortex. The surface layer, called the *molecular layer* in Fig. 6-12, is separated from the lowest layer, the *granular layer*, by a *layer of Purkinje cells*. The molecular layer and the granular layer get their names from their finely punctate and granular appearances, respectively, when a fresh section is cut through the cortex. The Purkinje cells, which lie between the two layers, are large neurons with dendrites branching far into the molecular layer. The Purkinje cell has already been shown in Fig. 1-3c. Apart from the Purkinje cells, the two other principal cell types in the cerebellar cortex are the *granule cells* in the granular layer and the *basket cells* in the molecular layer. The cerebellar cortex thus contains a total of three principal cell types.

Two types of axons (fibers) enter the cerebellar cortex. One of these, shown in Fig. 6-12A, is called a *climbing fiber*. It runs through the granular layer and ends in the molecular layer on the dendrites of the Purkinje cells. The ramifications of the climbing fibers "climb" up the dendritic tree and wrap themselves like ivy around the dendrites. The other fiber type is called a *mossy fiber* (Fig. 6-12B), and it terminates in the granular layer on the granule cells whose axons run between the Purkinje cells into the molecular layer where they divide up in T-shape fashion into two axon collaterals. The axons of the

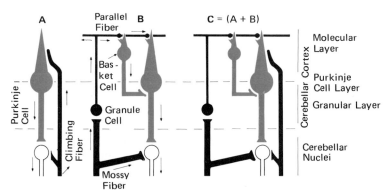

Fig. 6-12.   The most important neuronal circuits of the cerebellum. *A*: Synaptic connections of the climbing fibers. *B*: Synaptic connections of the mossy fibers. *C*: The afferent inputs of a Purkinje cell from the mossy and the climbing fibers. See this section for a detailed discussion of the anatomical connections and sec. 6.5 for a discussion of the function.

granule cells are called *parallel fibers* (in cross section they look like small dots or "molecules"). The parallel fibers are 2 to 3 mm long, and each fiber forms synapses on several dozen to several hundred *dendrites* of two types of cell: the basket cells and the Purkinje cells. The *basket cells*, in turn, send back their axons to the *soma* of the Purkinje cells. The mossy fibers thus do not reach the Purkinje cells directly (like the climbing fibers) but via one or two interneurons, the granule cells and the basket cells.

Only the axons of the Purkinje cells run from the cerebellar cortex to the neurons of the cerebellar nuclei. In addition, these cerebellar nuclear neurons receive collaterals of the climbing fibers (Fig. 6-12A) and the mossy fibers (Fig. 6-12B). In summary, the cerebellar cortex has two "inputs," the mossy fibers and the climbing fibers, and one "output," the axons of the Purkinje cells. All the information processing performed by the cerebellar cortex is carried out in neuronal networks such as the one illustrated in Fig. 6-12C (this is a collation of Fig. 6-12A and B). Altogether, the human cerebellar cortex contains about 15 million Purkinje cells. Each of these receives synapses from only a single climbing fiber but from many thousand parallel fibers and several dozen basket cells. The function of the cerebellar cortex is determined by the links between these pathways, the excitatory or the inhibitory polarity of the synapses, and the temporal sequence of the synaptic potentials and the action potentials. The most important details will be given in Sec. 6.5.

Now check your new knowledge.

Q 6.11 Which of the following structures has/have chiefly a motor function?
   a. Thalamus.
   b. Gyrus postcentralis.
   c. Sulcus centralis.
   d. Pallidum.
   e. Dorsal horn of the spinal cord.

Q 6.12 The pyramidal tract
   a. is only relayed in the brain stem.
   b. crosses 75 to 90 percent to the contralateral side.
   c. originates mainly in the Gyrus postcentralis.
   d. ends predominantly on spinal interneurons.
   e. is also called the Tractus corticospinalis.

Q 6.13 Which of the following statements is/are incorrect?
   a. An interruption of the motor pathways in the internal capsule leads to motor disturbances (paralysis) in the half of the body opposite the lesion.
   b. Extrapyramidal efferent axons originating in the motor cortex terminate at the latest in the brain stem.

    c. The Gyrus praecentralis is somatotopically organized; that is, certain areas serve certain peripheral muscles or groups of muscles.

    d. All the extrapyramidal pathways originating from the brain stem remain ipsilateral.

Q 6.14 The *dendrites* of the Purkinje cells of the cerebellum receive synapses from the
    a. parallel fibers of the granule cells.
    b. mossy fibers.
    c. climbing fibers.
    d. axons of the basket cells.

Q 6.15 The following axons form afferent "inputs" to the cerebellar cortex:
    a. Mossy fibers.
    b. Parallel fibers.
    c. Purkinje cell axons.
    d. Climbing fibers.

6.4 Reflex Control of the Body's Posture in Space

This section describes the capabilities of the motor centers of the brain stem. These can be analyzed experimentally by transecting the connections of the brain stem with the higher motor centers, that is, with the basal ganglia and the cerebral cortex, and perhaps also by removing the cerebellum. Along with such complete transections, more isolated stimulation and circumscribed lesion experiments have contributed to our knowledge of the motor centers of the brain stem. It has been discovered that these centers in the brain stem are responsible mainly for the reflex control of the body's position in space. To perform this task these brain stem centers evaluate the afferent information from a great many receptors in the body. Of particular importance here are the receptors of the vestibular organs (located bilaterally in the inner ears), the stretch receptors of the neck muscles, and the joint receptors in the region of the cervical vertebrae. With their help the motor centers of the brain stem are able to adjust and to maintain the normal body posture continuously and without any conscious control.

The sections of the brain stem and their afferent inputs.   The gray-shaded portions of the CNS shown in longitudinal section in Fig. 6-13 are termed collectively the *brain stem*. In the caudal direction the brain stem merges into the spinal cord. In the rostral (cranial) direc-

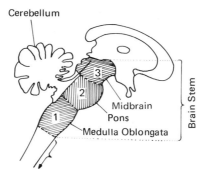

Fig. 6-13. Anatomical location of the most important parts of the brain stem. See text for details.

tion it joins up with the diencephalon, which contains the sensory nuclei of the thalamus (see Sec. 7.3), and the hypothalamus with important centers for the autonomic (vegetative) nervous system (see Sec. 8.5). In the direction from caudal to cranial we can distinguish histologically, phylogenetically, and, to some extent, also functionally three different sections of the brain stem: *medulla oblongata, pons,* and *midbrain.* The motor centers located cranially from the brain stem are the basal ganglia and the motor cortex (cf. Fig. 6-8 and 6-9). They transmit their information along the extrapyramidal pathways to the brain stem (cf. Fig. 6-11). Apart from these, there are additional important inputs for the motor centers of the brain stem. They are summarized in Fig. 6-14 as the impulses from receptors in the body's periphery (from skin, muscles, and joints), the cerebellum, and finally the vestibular organ.

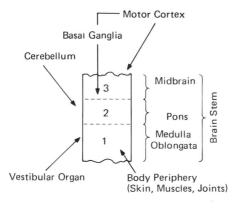

Fig. 6-14. Afferent and efferent inputs into the motor centers of the brain stem. Numbers 1 to 3 denote the sections of the brain stem identified by the same numbers in Fig. 6-13.

The *vestibular organ* is located directly alongside the auditory apparatus of the inner ear. Both are served by a common cranial nerve, the Nervus statoacusticus. The cavities of both organs intercommunicate. Anatomically they are very complex structures, and it is for this reason that they are referred to jointly as the labyrinth. The labyrinth is completely embedded in the temporal bone and is therefore not readily accessible either experimentally or surgically. The vestibular organ provides us with information about the position of our head in space (which we can state very accurately even with eyes shut and in the absence of any other reference points), as well as with information on angular acceleration (turning) and linear acceleration (in a car or in an elevator). Both positive and negative accelerations are indicated. The vestibular organ is somewhat sluggish in its responses. Thus, sensations often persist when an acceleration has ceased, as, for example, when a person comes to a sudden stop after turning around for some time. When the eyes are opened the CNS is supplied with contradictory afferent information from two different sources. Subjectively this gives rise to sensations of vertigo, or giddiness, and the objective result is disrupted motor coordination.

Transections in the brain stem. The influences of the motor centers located cranially from the brain stem, that is, the basal ganglia and the cerebral cortex, can be eliminated by making a transection at the upper boundary of the brain stem. (To be absolutely certain about the completeness of the transection the brain tissue on the rostral side of the transection site is usually completely removed). Such an animal is called a *midbrain animal* (Fig. 6-15A), because the midbrain is the highest still intact section of the CNS. If the transection is made a little lower down, say at the boundary between the midbrain and the pons, the animal is called a *decerebrate* animal (Fig. 6-15B). In this animal only the medulla oblongata and the pons are connected with the body by the spinal cord. Both the midbrain animal and the decerebrate animal have the same afferent connections. The cerebellar connections are also retained. Elimination of the latter does not appreciably affect the motor behavior of such animals.

Motor functions of the decerebrate animal; tonic neck reflexes. When the spinal cord is transected (spinalization, paraplegia) the peripheral musculature is either completely flaccid, or the tonus of the flexors predominates. Neither a person suffering from paraplegia nor a spinal animal can stand (see Sec. 6.2). On the other hand, in the decerebrate animal we find a strong increase in the tonus of the entire extensor musculature. As a result, the animal holds all four limbs in

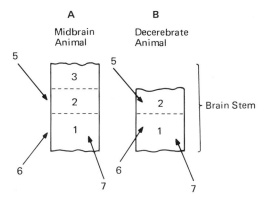

Fig. 6-15. Diagram showing the sections of the brain stem still connected to the body in a midbrain animal (*A*) and a decerebrate animal (*B*). The central and the peripheral inputs important for the motor system are also shown. Numbers 1 to 3 are the same as in Figs. 6-13 and 6-14 and denote the same sections of the brain stem. The afferents inputs correspond to those in Fig. 6-14, (5) cerebellum, (6) vestibular organ, and (7) body periphery.

the maximum extended position. Head and tail are bent toward the back. This particular group of symptoms is called *decerebrate rigidity*. If a decerebrate animal is stood upright, it remains standing since the joints do not bend as a result of the high degree of tonus of the extensor muscles. This unnatural overstretched posture of the animal seems like a caricature of normal standing. Since the decerebrate animal can stand, but the spinal animal cannot, it can be concluded that the medulla oblongata and the pons contain motor centers that control the muscle tone of the limbs in such a way that these can bear the weight of the body. The strongly increased extensor tone in the decerebrate animal indicates that these centers are disinhibited by the elimination of higher sections of the brain.

The distribution of tone in the musculature of a decerebrate animal can be varied by passive movement of the head. Since movements of the head vary its position both in space and relative to the body, this change in tone can be triggered by messages from the vestibular organ and/or receptors of the neck muscles. It is therefore necessary to study the changes in tone after one or the other of the sources of information has been eliminated. For example, if both labyrinths are removed, there is no longer information about the position of the head in space. However, the receptors of the neck musculature and the joints of the cervical vertebral column will signal each change in position of the head relative to the body. In the motor centers of the brain stem these signals generate corresponding and appropriate corrections in the distribution of muscle tone in the body musculature. We will now study some examples of such "tonic neck reflexes."

If the head of a decerebrate standing animal (labyrinths removed) is extended upward (red arrow in Fig. 6-16*A*), the tone of the limb muscles changes as shown: the extensor tone of the hind limb decreases and that of the fore limb increases. When the head is flexed (red arrow in Fig. 6-16*B*) exactly the opposite changes in the distribution of muscle tone occur: the extensor tone of the fore limbs decreases and that of the hind limbs increases. As a third example, if the head is turned to the side, that is, if the postural equilibrium is upset, this is compensated for by a corresponding change in tone of the musculature of the limbs. When the head is turned to the right (and the weight of the body is thus shifted to the right) the extensor tone of both right limbs increases. In all three cases the new posture is held for as long as the head remains in the changed position. These reflexes are therefore called *tonic neck reflexes.*

Tonic reflexes can be triggered by not only the receptors of the neck muscles but also by the labyrinths (no examples are given here). These summate with the neck reflexes when both information sources are intact. Thus the motor centers in the medulla oblongata and the pons are not only able to maintain sufficient tone in the limb muscles to keep the body standing against the force of gravity (decerebrate rigidity), but they can also modify this extreme extensor tone in accordance with the signals from the neck muscles and the labyrinths.

Decerebrate Animal with
Labyrinths removed

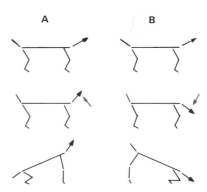

Fig. 6-16. Triggering of tonic neck reflexes in a decerebrate animal whose vestibular organs (labyrinths) have been removed. Passive stretching of the head upward (red arrow in *A*) results in a reduction in extensor tone in the hind limbs and an increase in extensor tone in the fore limbs. Passive flexing of the head (red arrow in *B*) has the opposite effect.

The changes in tone of the limb muscles brought about by changes in the position of the head are called *tonic neck and labyrinthine reflexes*.

An interesting special case among the tonic reflexes is that of the compensatory eye adjustments. These movements of the eyeballs ensure that the fields of vision remain the same even when the head moves. In man and animals with frontal eyes this is attained, for the most part, through the optical information derived from the overlapping fields of vision, but in animals with laterally arranged eyes, where the fields of vision of both eyes overlap only slightly or not at all, the distribution of the eye muscle tone is controlled largely by the interaction of tonic labyrinthine and neck reflexes. For example, if one turns the head of a rabbit so that the right half of the face moves downward, then the right eye is deflected upward and the left eye (the higher of the two) is deflected downward. The effect of this, to a certain extent at least, is that the eyes do not follow the position of the head but retain their position relative to the horizon.

Motor functions of the midbrain animal; righting reflexes. A decerebrate animal remains standing when it is placed upright on its legs, but it falls over when pushed and does not pick itself up again. Furthermore, the muscle tone is abnormal due to the strong predominance of extensor tone, whereas in normal standing the flexors and the extensors are activated approximately uniformly to fix a joint. If, in addition to the medulla oblongata and the pons, the midbrain is also left in contact with the spinal cord, then the motor capabilities of the animal are considerably expanded and improved. The two most noticeable differences between a midbrain and a decerebrate animal are: (1) the midbrain animal exhibits no decerebrate rigidity; that is, the preferential activation of the extensor muscles no longer occurs. (2) The midbrain animal can *stand up* by itself. As Fig. 6-15 shows, the relevant motor inputs into the brain stem of the midbrain animal are no different from those of the decerebrate animal; therefore the improvements in the motor functions of the midbrain animal compared with those of the decerebrate animal must be determined predominantly by the motor centers of the midbrain.

The missing decerebrate rigidity in the case of the normally standing midbrain animal indicates that the distribution of tone in the flexors and the extensors of this animal is more physiological than in the decerebrate animal. More important than the missing decerebrate rigidity is the ability of the midbrain animal to attain the standing or the upright posture. From all other positions, the basic standing position is in each case assumed in a reflex manner and with complete reliability.

The reflexes that bring about this adoption of the upright posture are called *righting reflexes*. It has been found that the righting reflexes governing the adoption of the normal upright posture occur in a certain set sequence, or a chain of reflexes. To start with, the head is always brought to the normal position in accordance with information received from the labyrinths (vestibular organs). These reflexes are called *labyrinthine righting reflexes*. Raising of the head when the animal is lying down, for example, changes the position of the head relative to the rest of the body, and this is indicated by the receptors of the neck muscles. The signals from the receptors of the neck musculature cause the trunk to follow the head into the normal position. In the same way that the righting reflexes originating from the labyrinth are called labyrinthine righting reflexes, those issuing from the neck muscles are referred to as *neck righting reflexes*.

Righting reflexes are thus reflexes that bring the body back to the normal upright position. As a result of these reflexes the normal posture and state of equilibrium of the body are maintained without conscious control. Besides those mentioned, there are a whole series of righting reflexes that originate, for example, from the receptors of the body's surface and act upon the position of head and body. If one also includes here the optical righting reflexes, which are eliminated in the midbrain animal, but which can be detected under other experimental conditions, then it becomes clear that the righting of the body that can be triggered in so many different ways is one of the most reliable functions of the CNS. Through the tonic and the righting reflexes it is guaranteed that the body can take up and maintain a basic upright posture. It is important that in these reactions the major role is played by the head, which contains the eyes, the ears, and the nose. Because of this the body can adopt a suitable posture—frequently a defensive posture—when it senses stimuli from still far-off sources.

The reflexes described so far are often grouped together under the category *static* reflexes because they control and maintain the attitude and the balance of the body when it is lying, standing, or sitting quietly in various positions. In addition, a number of reflexes can be detected in the midbrain animal that are induced by motion, and these are therefore called *statokinetic* reflexes. Many of these originate in the labyrinth. The best known are the reactions of the eyes and the head to rotation. For example, if an animal is turned in a clockwise direction the head turns in an anticlockwise direction, and so on. These reactions are compensatory; that is, the eyes and the head move in such a way that the fixation of the eyes is maintained as far as possible during the motion. Once the movement has stopped the eye positions are held by static reflexes (compensatory eye adjustments;

see above). Other important statokinetic reflexes ensure balance and correct posture when the animal jumps or runs. These reflexes, for example, enable a cat always to land the right way up regardless of the position from which it is dropped.

On the whole it can be said that as regards the tonic, the righting, the running, and the jumping reactions there is scarcely any difference between the midbrain animal and the intact animal. However, the midbrain animal is incapable of spontaneous movement, and in each case an external stimulus is required before the animal, which behaves like a robot, will move. The experiments on decerebrate and midbrain animals show without doubt that the various extremely expressive postures and attitudes of animals and man, which we encounter in our normal existence as well as in painting and sculpture, are based in the final analysis on the laws governing the motor centers of the brain stem and their integration of the sequence of righting and tonic reflexes. These reflexes cause all the muscles of the body to act together to assume or to maintain a desired attitude.

Please work through the following questions to check whether you have assimilated the material contained in this section.

Q 6.16 Which portions of the brain stem remain in contact with the spinal cord in the decerebrate animal; that is, which are still functional?
  a. Medulla oblongata
  b. Pons and midbrain.
  c. Medulla oblongata and pons.
  d. Medulla oblongata and midbrain.
  e. Medulla oblongata, pons, and midbrain.

Q 6.17 Which of the multiple-choice answers given in question 6.16 includes all the intact brain stem regions of the midbrain animal?

Q 6.18 Which of the following characteristics are *not* possessed by the decerebrate animal?
  a. Decerebrate rigidity.
  b. Righting reflexes.
  c. Predominance of extensor tonus.
  d. Tonic reflexes.
  e. Predominance of flexor tonus.

Q 6.19 The motor centers of the midbrain animal have the same afferent inputs as the motor centers of the decerebrate animal. Which two sources of input listed below are particularly important for the tonic and the righting reflexes?
  a. Cerebellum.
  b. Vestibular organ of the labyrinth.
  c. Receptors of the body surface.

    d. Muscle and the joint receptors of the body.

    e. Muscle and the joint receptors of the neck.

Q 6.20 Which of the following tonic and righting reflexes have afferents in the labyrinth, and which have them in the neck muscles?

    a. Increase of extensor tonus of fore limbs when raising the head.

    b. Decrease of extensor tonus of left limbs when the head is rotated to the right.

    c. Raising of the body to the normal upright position.

    d. Raising of the head to the normal upright position.

6.5   Motor Functions of the Cerebrum and the Cerebellum

In our analysis of the central nervous structures important for the motor capabilities of the body, we come now to a discussion of the function of the motor areas of the cerebrum and their associated basal ganglia and the tasks of the cerebellum. Here, as everywhere in the CNS, there are two main questions to answer: (1) what do these centers do? and (2) how do they do it? We will only be able to give very incomplete answers because, first, our knowledge of what these centers do, and still more so of how they do it, is in many respects very sketchy; second, we are restricting ourselves in this book to the essential and experimentally well-documented fundamentals of neurophysiology. But, particularly in the discussion of the higher motor functions it is understandable, in view of the complexity of the subject, that a greal deal of hypothesis and speculation should go hand in hand with scientifically established fact. Therefore, in this section, we shall begin by studying the tasks of the motor areas of the cerebrum and the associated basal ganglia without considering how these tasks are achieved. Then the functions of the cerebellum will be discussed, and we shall also examine, at least in broad outline, how the cerebellum processes its information.

Performance of the motor cortex; decorticate animal.   If the entire cerebral cortex is removed from an animal it is called a *decorticate animal*. Compared with an intact animal the decorticate animal exhibits three important motor defects: (1) a series of complex reflex patterns of movement is missing (no examples given here); (2) all acquired motor capabilities are lost; and (3) spontaneous and voluntary motor functions disappear completely (animal behaves like a robot). The disappearance of these reflexes permits us to conclude that certain congenital reflex patterns of movement are programmed in the cerebral cortex and that the cortex is involved in more than just voluntary motor functions. The loss of all acquired motor capabilities demonstrates that only the cortex is properly in a position to store and to convert information into purposeful motor behavior patterns. The significance of the complete loss of spontaneous and voluntary motor functions becomes clearer if only the motor areas of the cerebral cortex of an animal are lesioned while the rest of the cerebral cortex remains intact. Such an animal also behaves like a robot. This indicates that the motor expression of any CNS activity localized in the cerebral cortex (and that includes all the higher abilities of the CNS) takes place through the motor cortex and cannot reach the subcortical motor centers directly from the relevant cortical areas.

The most important motor area of the brain is the *Gyrus praecentralis* situated in front of the Sulcus centralis. It is connected mainly with the motoneurons of the contralateral half of the body by the pyramidal tract and, to some extent, also by the extrapyramidal pathways. Other motor areas are located in the vicinity of the Gyrus praecentralis, mainly frontally from it (toward the forehead). While the pyramidal tract originates chiefly but not exclusively from the Gyrus praecentralis, the extrapyramidal pathways originate primarily but not exclusively from the other motor areas. The Gyrus praecentralis is somatotopically organized while the other motor areas do not exhibit any pronounced somatotopic organization.

Tasks of the pyramidal tract and the extrapyramidal pathways. As we have learned, the pyramidal tract projects without relaying into the spinal cord, while the extrapyramidal pathways are relayed several times. The pyramidal tract thus possesses more direct access to the motoneurons. In keeping with this differentiation, the two descending systems also have *different tasks* to perform. *The pyramidal tract serves mainly to permit rapid voluntary motion.* Its axons act on the α motoneurons to some extent directly, but for the most part through segmental interneurons. On the whole, a *facilitatory* influence of the pyramidal tract on the α motoneurons predominates. Isolated lesions of the pyramidal tract thus will tend to bring about a *flaccid* paralysis. The *extrapyramidal pathways* originating from the cerebral cortex *serve primarily to control postural functions* (slow movements, adjustment of tonus). On the whole there is a predominant *inhibitory* influence of the extrapyramidal corticofugal pathways on the subcortical motor centers and consequently on the motoneurons. Isolated lesion of these pathways will tend to produce *spastic* paralysis.

As already described in the discussion of segmental reflexes, a change in muscle tonus can be brought about by direct facilitatory and inhibitory influences acting on the α motoneurons of the extrafusal muscle fibers, and by activation or depression of the monosynaptic stretch reflex via the γ motoneurons that innervate the intrafusal muscle fibers of the muscle spindles. The first way is faster; the second has the advantage of more precisely graduated control (Sec. 6.1). It has been found that the axons of the pyramidal tract act mainly on the α motoneurons, bypassing the γ loop, while the extrapyramidal pathways end preferentially on γ motoneurons; that is, they operate through the γ loop and thus through the reflex arc of the monosynaptic stretch reflex. With regard to the tasks just described for the two efferent systems, this arrangement would appear to be extremely advantageous.

The axons of the *corticofugal* extrapyramidal neurons are relayed at the latest in the brain stem (Fig. 6-11). Lesion of these corticofugal pathways increases the muscle tone because, as seen above, taken as a whole their inhibitory influence on the α motoneurons predominates. To put this more precisely: the motor centers of the brain stem, which are part of the extrapyramidal motor system, on the whole exert a predominantly facilitatory influence on the segmental motoneurons. However, under normal circumstances these centers are under the mainly inhibitory control of the corticofugal neurons. Elimination of this control then leads to increased muscle tone. This is certainly a part of the mechanism of decerebrate rigidity.

Figure 6-17 summarizes the most important afferent, efferent, and intercortical connections of the cortical motor areas: the descending pathways of the extrapyramidal motor system and the pyramidal tract are shown in red. All details of the other connections of the motor cortex with other cortical areas and the sense organs have been left out, but it must be stressed that these connections are very important for the proper functioning of the motor cortex. All motor centers have a large number of afferent inputs that supply them from the environment and from within the body with the information they need to carry out their tasks and that make it possible for them to coordinate their activity with that of other motor centers. We have seen, for example, that in the case of the tonic and the righting reflexes the most important sources of information, along with the visual inputs, are the vestibular organ and the neck muscle afferents. As already seen in Fig. 6-8, the cerebellum is connected in parallel with the other motor centers. However, it is connected with *all* the afferent and the efferent pathways. The cerebellum transmits its efferent messages directly to the cortical motor centers and also (red arrow in Fig. 6-17) to the

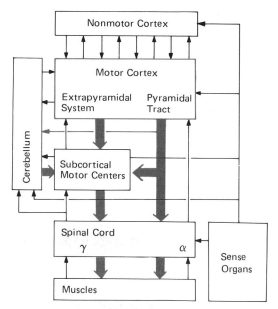

Fig. 6-17. Block diagram of the connections of the cortical motor centers with the other motor centers, the rest of the cortex, the cerebellum, the muscles, and the sense organs.

subcortical motor centers of the extrapyramidal system. Thus, because of its connections, the cerebellum seems particularly well able to coordinate the activity of the various motor centers.

Motor disturbances deriving from clinical disorders. Let us now apply our knowledge to disorders of the cortical motor centers. Lesions of the left Gyrus praecentralis will result in paralysis in the right half of the body. The site and the extent of the damage determine the localization and the severity of the paralysis. For example, injury in the lateral-caudal part of the Gyrus praecentralis will paralyze the face muscles. However, rather than direct damage to the Gyrus praecentralis, a much more frequent clinical finding is interruption of the descending pathways, particularly in the region of the internal capsule (Capsula interna) where the pyramidal tract and parts of the extrapyramidal pathway emerge between the basal ganglia and the thalamus (Figs. 6-10 and 6-11). Sudden hemorrhaging or thromboses in this area give rise to the group of symptoms characterizing a stroke. Because of the descending pathways that are involved, there are symptoms of both pyramidal and extrapyramidal lesions. The contralateral half of the body is always paralyzed (hemiplegia). The paralysis is, above all, a symptom of damage to the pyramidal tract. During the initial stage of shock the paralysis is flaccid. However, once this initial stage recedes, the paralysis usually becomes spastic, that is, the paralyzed muscles exhibit a high degree of tone. This high degree of muscle tone on the paralyzed side of the body is chiefly a symptom of lesion of the extrapyramidal pathways. In severe cases; the clincial picture is reminiscent of experimentally produced decerebrate rigidity.

Phylogenetic differences in the importance of the motor centers; the role of the basal ganglia.   It should now be mentioned briefly that the behavioral patterns described so far for midbrain and also decorticate animals, strictly speaking, apply only to certain mammals, especially rabbits, cats, and dogs. In the lower vertebrates, such as birds, the deficits are, in general, less severe, but in the higher mammals, particularly in the primates, they are usually more pronounced. In the latter animals and in man the increase in motor capabilities has been accompanied by an ever greater shift of the motor control functions toward the cortex (cephalization). Nevertheless, it is true to say that in primates, including man, the individual motor centers still retain their assigned functions within the overall control framework of the motor system: they are simply no longer able to function at maximum or near maximum efficiency without their connections to the next higher centers.

A typical example of these processes is supplied by the phylogenetic fate of the basal ganglia. These are the highest motor centers in birds and other low vertebrates, and these animals have very little cortical substance. In the higher vertebrates, particularly man, the functions of the basal ganglia have been shifted toward the cortex at the same time that a great increase has occurred in the volume of the cerebral cortex, and the role of the basal ganglia is no longer so clearly defined. In the basal ganglia we can distinguish, primarily on the basis of phylogenetic, histological, and clinical evidence, the *striatum*, which is made up of the N. caudatus and putamen, and the *pallidum*, which consists of an outer and an inner part (for their anatomical position in the brain see Figs. 6-9, 6-10, and 6-11). In addition, two nuclei situated in the midbrain, N. ruber and N. niger, are included in the basal ganglia, but functionally they belong to the brain stem centers that have already been discussed. In man, damage to the basal ganglia leads to motor disorders with excessive movement (chorea, athetosis) when the striatum is affected and to tremor (trembling), rigidity (muscular tension), and hypokinesia when the pallidum is affected (grouped together these latter symptoms are called

Parkinson's syndrome). Similar motor derangements can be detected in animals, particularly in primates, when the striatum or the pallidum is damaged. From these findings it can be concluded that the basal ganglia in man are chiefly responsible for the smooth and proper implementation of voluntary movements.

Role of the cerebellum; lesion symptoms.   Let us now look at the tasks the *cerebellum* has to perform. Anatomically, the cerebellum consists of the cerebellar cortex and the cerebellar nuclei. The macroscopic structure of the individual lobes of the cortex and the connections of the various parts of the cortex with the individual cerebellar nuclei will not be discussed further here. We shall go into neither the phylogenetic origin of the various lobes of the cerebellum nor the fact that the cerebellum is to a certain extent somatotopically organized. It is not strictly necessary to know all this in order to understand the most important functions of the cerebellum as they are described here.

It has already been mentioned in connection with Figs. 6-8 and 6-17 that the cerebellum is connected in parallel with the other motor centers. In addition, the cerebellum receives afferent messages from practically all the sense organs. From these findings the conclusion was drawn above that the cerebellum appears particularly well suited to coordinate the activity of the various motor centers with one another. This assumption is supported by experimental and clincial findings. It has been found that the cerebellum is above all required for the smooth, purposeful implementation of the voluntary movements "planned" by the cerebrum, as well as for the coordination of these voluntary movements with the involuntary motor activities that serve to control muscular tone, posture, and equilibrium. It follows that if the cerebellum is damaged or destroyed, the functional derangements are most apparent when the patient is moving.

When the cerebellum is completely disrupted three symptoms appear: (1) *ataxia*—a stumbling, staggering gait because the muscular contractions needed for movement do not occur at the right moment and to the right degree; (2) *adiadochokinesia*—the inability to perform rapid alternating movements (piano playing); and (3) *intention tremor*—a trembling that occurs during the execution of purposeful voluntary movement. When the cerebellum is completely disrupted, individual motor capabilities (for instance, tonic reflexes) do not fail, but instead there are malfunctions in the coordination of the motor centers that are apparent in the three symptoms just mentioned. When the cerebellum is only partially out of action the motor derangements are correspondingly less pronounced or limited to certain areas (for example, just in one arm) or movements.

The cerebellum is thus like the computer in a factory. It calculates the flow of parts and materials along the various production lines in such a way that, when all the components come together at the final assembly stage, there are no bottlenecks or gaps in the flow. To achieve this, the computer needs a continuous feedback regarding the production status at any one time. The cerebellum also requires continuous feedback information on all the movements occurring at any one time if it is to accomplish its task properly.

Figure 6-18 shows the most important feedback circuits to the cerebellum. The pyramidal tract puts out axonal collaterals to the cerebellum so that the cerebellum is kept informed about voluntary movement *in advance*. Because of this advance report from the pyramidal tract the cerebellum can suitably modify the excitatory flux in the extrapyramidal motor system (for example, shift the balance) and also influence voluntary movements while they are occurring by means of feedback to the motor cortex. Apart from these advance reports, the cerebellum receives continuous feedback from the entire sensory system on the course of the voluntary and the involuntary movements. It is therefore able to make corrections in good time so

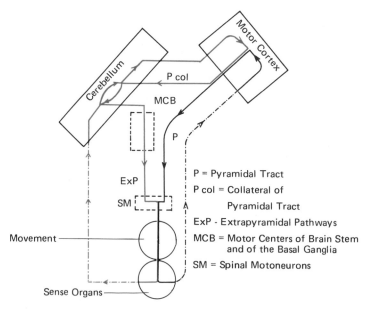

Fig. 6-18.   Diagram of the most important feedback circuits to the cerebellum. See text for details.

that, for example, voluntary movements can be carried out without visible deviation from their goal, that is, without intention tremor.

Circuits in the cerebellar cortex. Let us now look briefly at the question of how the cerebellum performs its function. The flow diagram of the cerebellar inputs and outputs in Fig. 6-19 shows that the cerebellar cortex possesses two inputs, the mossy fibers and the climbing fibers, and one output, the Purkinje cell axons, as we have already discussed in Sec. 6.3. The cerebellar nuclei connect the cerebellum with the other motor centers. Information is processed by the cerebellum mainly in the cortex. The diagram of one complete neuronal circuit from the cerebellum (there are many millions of such circuits) is shown in Fig. 6-12*C*. In this circuit diagram, or on a copy, insert the names of the individual components and indicate the flow direction of the axonal impulses as in Fig. 6-12*A* and *B*. The polarity of the synapses is indicated by the color of the individual components: black axons form excitatory and red axons inhibitory synapses.

The *climbing fibers* thus form excitatory synapses on the dendrites of the Purkinje cells. The actions of the *mossy fibers* are more complex. They excite the granule cells whose parallel fibers in turn have an excitatory effect on the basket cells and the Purkinje cells. It is interesting to note, however, that the basket cells inhibit the Purkinje

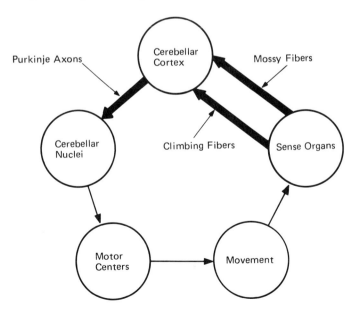

Fig. 6-19. Flow diagram of cerebellar inputs and outputs. See text for details.

cells. The parallel fibers (and thus the mossy fibers) therefore have a double action on the Purkinje cells: excitatory on the dendrites and inhibitory on the soma via the basket cells. This inhibition of the Purkinje cells by the basket cells is a typical example of *feed-forward inhibition.* In contrast to feedback inhibition, the inhibition occurs regardless of whether or not the inhibited cell was excited beforehand (cf. in this connection Fig. 4-4*B*). Since the inhibitory synapse of the basket cell is located on the axon hillock it is likely to be particularly effective. Finally, the Purkinje cell axons form inhibitory synapses on the cells of the cerebellar nuclei. Since the Purkinje cells discharge spontaneously, a change in the Purkinje cell output is reflected in either an increase in these discharges (that is, increased inhibition of cells in the cerebellar nuclei) or in a decrease in the discharges (removal of inhibition of these cells = disinhibition).

Under resting conditions the Purkinje cell discharges will thus lead to tonic inhibition of the cerebellar nuclei. Afferent activity of the climbing fibers increases this inhibition because these fibers excite the Purkinje cells. Afferent activity in the mossy fibers, on the other hand, may exert a dual effect: excitation by the parallel fibers and inhibition by the basket cells. It is still not completely clear which sensory modalities or which of their parameters are transmitted by the mossy fibers and which by the climbing fibers. Likewise, the connection patterns of the parallel fibers are still not known well enough, even though it has been discovered that mossy fiber activity usually leads to excitation of defined groups of Purkinje cells while neighboring Purkinje cells are inhibited.

The physiology of the cerebellum can be taken as an example of how far research into the physiology of the brain has progressed in answering the "what" and "why" questions of central nervous activity. Despite all our detailed knowledge of cerebellar circuits and their inputs and outputs, we still cannot explain with much more precision how these circuits accomplish the cerebellar functions that have been outlined. More thought and more experiments are needed before this unsatisfactory situation can be remedied. The progress made in the past decades in many areas of neurophysiology gives us cause to hope that we will soon achieve new and decisive breakthroughs in our knowledge of central nervous activity. In any event, there seems no reason right now to believe, as is sometimes claimed, that the brain is unable to "understand itself."

Please work through the following steps to check whether you have remembered all these facts about the motor centers of the cerebrum and the cerebellum.

Q 6.21 In a decorticate animal, which of the following motor functions are extinguished?
   a. Voluntary motor functions.
   b. Tonic reflexes.
   c. Righting reflexes.
   d. Acquired motor functions.
   e. Flexor reflexes.

Q 6.22 Where are the cells of origin of the pyramidal tract located?
   a. Exclusively in the Gyrus postcentralis.
   b. In the Gyrus postcentralis and in the neighboring parietal areas.
   c. In the basal ganglia, particularly in the pallidum.
   d. Exclusively in the Gyrus praecentralis.
   e. In the Gyrus praecentralis and in the neighboring frontal areas.
   f. All the foregoing statements are false.

Q 6.23 Which of the following statements about the pyramidal tract are correct?
   a. It runs with one relay in the basal nuclei right into the spinal cord.
   b. It serves chiefly to transmit rapid voluntary movements.
   c. Its axons mainly end directly on the motoneurons.
   d. It activates mostly α motoneurons via interneurons.
   e. Unilateral selective lesion of the pyramidal tract above the medulla oblongata leads to ipsilateral flaccid paralysis.

Q 6.24 Which of the following symptoms are characteristic of a simultaneous interruption of the pyramidal and the extrapyramidal pathways in the left inner capsule?
   a. Passive tremor.
   b. Intention tremor.
   c. Flaccid paralysis, left side.
   d. Adiadochokinesia.
   e. Parkinsonism, right side.
   f. None of the above symptoms is characteristic.

Q 6.25 Inhibitory synapses on the dendrites of the Purkinje cells of the cerebellum are formed by
   a. climbing fibers directly.
   b. mossy fibers via granule cells and parallel fibers.
   c. climbing fibers via basket cells.
   d. mossy fibers via granule cells and basket cells.
   e. all of the above.
   f. none of the above.

Q 6.26 Which of the following symptoms are characteristic of a cerebellar lesion?
  a. Passive tremor.
  b. Intention tremor.
  c. Athetosis.
  d. Adiadochokinesia.
  e. Ataxia.
  f. Parkinsonism.
  g. Hemiplegia.

7

SENSORY SYSTEM

The term "sensory system" is used to denote those parts of the nervous system that detect, transmit, and process messages from the environment and from inside the body. The sensory system is involved in practically all the functions of the nervous system, for example, control of the body's posture in space and maintenance of a constant body temperature. These two examples also show that sensory events in the nervous system are not necessarily consciously perceived. In fact, by far the greater part of these sensory events occur outside the realm of our conscious awareness.

This chapter provides a general introduction to the basic principles of the sensory functions of the nervous system, taking examples chiefly from the somatosensory system (= sensory system of the body surface, chiefly that of the skin). With a few exceptions, we will restrict ourselves to objective observations, that is, to neurophysiologically detectable events. The subjective sensory perceptions and the psychophysical correlations belong to the domain of sensory physiology. Sensory physiology also includes the neurophysiology of the special sense organs (eye, ear, and so on), and will be dealt with in a separate volume.

7.1 Transformation of Stimuli by Receptors

Adequate stimulus, classification of receptors. In the introduction to the structure of the nervous system (Chapter 1) a receptor was defined as a specialized nerve cell that informs the CNS about events occurring inside the body or in its environment. These events acting on the receptors are also known as *stimuli*. Stimuli have objectively measurable parameters such as temperature, mechanical deformation of the skin, or electromagnetic radiation (light). Physiological tests have shown that each receptor responds particularly readily to one form of stimulus. This characteristic is generally termed the *specificity* of the receptors, and the effective stimulus in each case is known as the *adequate stimulus*. Our everyday experience can provide us with evidence of the existence of such adequate stimuli for some of the body's receptors. It is not difficult to establish, for example, that the adequate stimulus for the receptors of our eyes is light, whereas we cannot perceive thermal or mechanical stimuli with these receptors. The adequate stimulus of individual receptors can be determined exactly in animal experiments. Each receptor is able to provide the CNS with information on only one particular aspect or section of the environment, and it may be said that it performs a *filter function*. Thus, in addition to the classification given earlier (see Sec. 1.1), it seems useful to classify the receptors on the basis of the adequate stimulus.

The receptors of mammals can be classified into four groups: *mechanoreceptors, thermoreceptors, chemoreceptors,* and *photoreceptors*. Among the mechanoreceptors, thermoreceptors, and probably also the chemoreceptors, there are some that respond only to very high stimulus intensity. These receptors presumably evoke pain sensations. Such receptors are also termed *nociceptors*. Within each group a still finer classification can be made, and the adequate stimulus is once more the criterion. For example, individual photoreceptors respond to light of different wavelengths (red, green, blue). In this case, the receptors are color-specific. The thermoreceptors can be subdivided into a group of warm receptors and a group of cold receptors. In other words, they respond, respectively, to a rise or a fall in temperature of the surrounding tissue relative to the normal body temperature. Mechanoreceptors are also specialized to respond to various mechanical stimulus parameters. There are, for example, receptors for high-frequency vibration and others for constant pressure.

The receptor potential.   A description will now be given of the events that take place in a receptor in response to an adequate stimulus and that lead to action potentials in the afferent fibers. The example that we shall use is that of the stretch receptor of the crayfish. This is a mechanoreceptor situated between the muscle fibers of the animals, and it responds to stretching of the muscle. The receptor corresponds in function to the muscle spindles of vertebrates. Compared with other receptors, this receptor is particularly large (about 100 μ in diameter), and it is therefore ideally suited for investigation by intracellular electrodes (Fig. 7-1).

When an intracellular microelectrode is inserted into the receptor

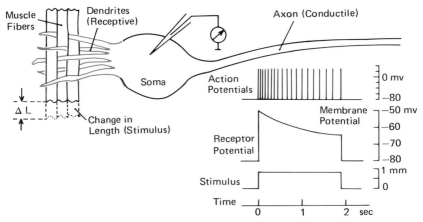

Fig. 7-1. Electrophysiological measurements taken at a stretch receptor (diagrammatic representation). During a stimulus (change in length of the surrounding muscle) the microelectrode records the receptor potential which is generated in the receptive region (dendrites). The receptor potential triggers propagated action potentials in the axon (conductile membrane).

a resting potential is recorded (-80 mV in Fig. 7-1). When an adequate stimulus is applied, that is, when the surrounding muscle is stretched, a depolarizing change in potential occurs. This stimulus-induced depolarization is called the *receptor potential*. The receptor potential in Fig. 7-1 lasts as long as the stimulus (stretch in Fig. 7-1). In the course of a constant stretch (square-wave stimulus), the receptor potential declines from an initial maximum (30 mV in Fig. 7-1) to a lower value. This decrease of the receptor potential in the course of a stimulus of constant intensity is observed in almost all receptors. The phenomenon is referred to as *adaptation*. We shall deal with this aspect of the receptor characteristics in more detail below.

The receptor potential is brought about by a nonspecific increase in membrane conductance for all small ions (Na^+, K^+, Ca^{++}, Cl^-). To induce depolarizations, for instance by about 30 mV, the ions flowing through the membrane must include some whose equilibrium potential is far from the resting potential in the depolarizing direction. Under normal conditions only Na^+ ions meet this requirement. Consequently, these ions must be the main factor in the generation of the receptor potential.

The increase in conductance at the receptors, which has just been described, is similar to that taking place at the subsynaptic membrane of excitatory synapses, for example, at the motor end plate (see Chapter 3).

The increase in conductance that brings about the receptor potential is localized in a specialized region of the receptor cell, namely, in the *receptive* membrane (shown in red in Fig. 7-1). It has been shown that stimuli evoke a receptor potential only if they are applied at this specialized region of the receptor cell. The receptive region of the membrane is thus different from the other parts of the cell, for example, the *conductile* membrane of the axon. A delineation is also possible by pharmacological means: the conductile membrane can be selectively poisoned by using, for example, TTX (tetrodotoxin) so that no further action potentials can be triggered here. The receptor potential, on the other hand, is not affected by TTX.

In the stretch receptor of the crayfish the receptive membrane is located close to the soma in the region of the dendrites. In contrast, the receptors of mammals are usually located at the most distal end of the axon. Because of their small size it has not been possible so far to record intracellularly the receptor potentials of these receptive endings. On stimulation, however, it is possible to record extracellular currents in the region of the receptor ending, which have been recognized to be generated by changes in membrane conductance for small ions. From this it can be concluded that at these receptors, too, a receptor potential occurs as an intermediate stage in stimulus transformation.

When we compare the stimulus energy acting on the receptor with the electrical energy of the receptor potential (product of change in potential and the electrical charge), we find that in many receptors a very considerable amplification takes place. For example, in a photoreceptor the electrical energy of the receptor potential may be more than 1,000 times as great as the energy of the light stimulus. It must be concluded therefore that the stimuli release locally stored energy. The intermediate stages from the impingement of a stimulus to the generation of the receptor potential, the so-called *primary transduction process*, have still not been investigated extensively.

It is assumed that subcellular structures (generally known as organelles) are also involved here. Such structures (for example, lamelliform organelles carrying light-sensitive pigment molecules in certain photoreceptors) have been discovered in the region of receptor endings, particularly with the aid of electron microscopy. These structures are presumed to have the function of auxiliary devices, which provide a receptor with the high degree of sensitivity for a particular form of stimulus, namely, the adequate stimulus in each case (specificity).

In many receptors the nerve ending is closely associated with a cell of nonneural origin whose morphological structure is also thought to be important for the specificity of a receptor (for example, the hair cells of the inner ear and the labyrinth whose long cilia are assumed to be sensors for extremely fine mechanical stimuli). These attempted explanations, however, should not hide the fact that practically nothing is known about the manner in which such structures participate in the primary transduction process.

The receptor potential as a generator of propagated action potentials. The receptor potential spreads electrotonically (see Chapter 2) to the adjacent areas of the cell. As a result, the axon is also depolarized. When this depolarization reaches the threshold of the axon membrane, an action potential is triggered. The action potential is conducted along the axon to the CNS. The receptor potential thus acts on the axon membrane as an electrical stimulus and is therefore also called the *generator potential*. When the receptor potential lasts beyond the end of the action potential, a further action potential can be triggered. Similarly, additional action potentials can occur until the stimulus and thus the receptor potential cease. During long-lasting receptor potentials the afferent fiber of the receptor discharges repetitively, as shown in Fig. 7-1.

The transformation of a stimulus into neuronal activity takes place as follows: acting via an unknown mechanism (primary transduction process) the stimulus brings about an increase in conductance for small ions. The resulting change in membrane potential is the receptor potential. This spreads electrotonically to the afferent axon, and when the threshold is reached it triggers one or more action potentials which are transmitted to the CNS.

In our discussion of the receptor potential we have already mentioned that the receptor potential decreases even when the stimulus remains constant with respect to time. This phenomenon, called *adaptation*, also occurs during the discharge sequence in the afferent nerve fibers. As indicated in Fig. 7-1, during the course of a stimulus the time interval Δt between two successive nerve pulses increases, or, to put it another way, the instantaneous frequency decreases (frequency = $1/\Delta t$).

If the responses of different receptors to suprathreshold square-wave stimuli are investigated, quite different time courses are found for the discharge frequency. Figure 7-2A shows the discharge of three receptors, one with slow (c), one with medium-fast (b), and one with very fast (a) adaptation. Figure 7-2B shows the time course of the instantaneous frequency for the slow and the medium-fast adapting receptors.

Adaptation should be interpreted not only as a fatigue phenomenon of the receptors, and consequently as an adverse factor. The

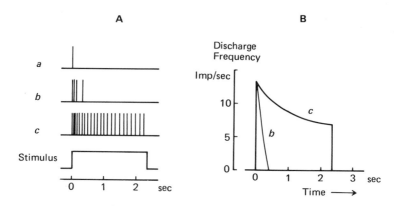

Fig. 7-2. Discharges of receptors having different adaptation rates. A: The action potentials of a very fast (*a*), a medium-fast (*b*) and a slow-adapting (*c*) receptor in the case of a long-duration, temporally constant stimulus. B: The time course of the instantaneous frequency during the stimulus for the last two receptor types (*b*, *c*).

decline in the discharge frequency during long-term stimulation can also be interpreted as an economy principle: few impulses per unit of time for the long-term signaling of a constant state means increased "impulse frequency reserves" to signal any changes in a state. This economy of information applies to both the transmission of data in the nerve fibers and the processing of the data in the CNS.

Control of receptor potential and discharge frequency by the stimulus intensity. If the receptor is stimulated by a series of stimuli of varying intensity, then the resulting receptor potentials also vary accordingly in magnitude or amplitude. This dependence of the receptor potential on the stimulus strength is shown in Fig. 7-3. Like the stimulus strength, the amplitude of the receptor potential also increases in Fig. 7-3A in the sequence *c*, *b*, *a*. The time course is the same for all three potentials. If the magnitude of the receptor potentials in Fig. 7-3A is measured at a fixed time, the relationship between stimulus strength and receptor potential can be expressed quantitatively, for example, in graph form as shown in Fig. 7-3B. In this diagram the circles denote measurements taken in the stretch receptor of a crayfish. The measurements lie along a straight line, and in this case the relationship between stimulus intensity, S, and receptor potential, R, is *linear*: $R = k \times S$ (k is a proportionality factor). The linear relationship is a special case. In other receptors the relationship is *nonlinear*, as, for example, in the photoreceptor of the compound eye of the horseshoe crab, *Limulus* (dotted curve in Fig. 7-3B).

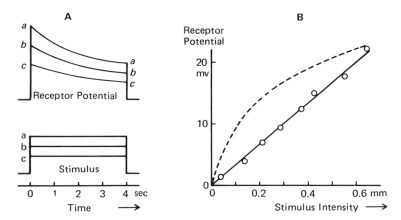

Fig. 7-3. Diagram of the relationship between stimulus intensity and receptor potential. The receptor potentials of a stretch receptor (top part of *A*) are shown for three stimuli of varying intensity (lower part of *A*). The quantitative relationship between the magnitude of the receptor potential at a given time during the stimulus and the stimulus intensity (= change in length of the stretch receptor) is shown in graph form in *B*. The dotted line in *B* shows, for the sake of comparison, a nonlinear relationship between the two parameters.

While the magnitude of the receptor potential depends continuously on the stimulus strength, the amplitude of each action potential generated in the receptor is independent of the stimulus strength. However, increasing stimulus strength brings about an increase in the *frequency* of the action potentials. These facts are represented in Fig. 7-4 for the stretch receptor. Three stimuli of varying intensity are

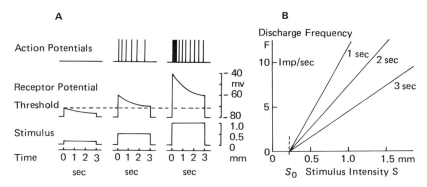

Fig. 7-4. Relationship between stimulus intensity and discharge frequency. *A*: Receptor potentials and action potentials for stimuli of various intensities. *B*: A graph of the instantaneous action potential frequency at three different times (1, 2, and 3 sec) after the start of the stimulus as a function of the stimulus intensity S. S_0 is the stimulus threshold.

shown from left to right in A, and above them in each case are given the receptor potential and the repetitive action potentials. The stimulus on the left does not trigger any action potential. Its receptor potential does not reach the depolarization threshold of the axon. As the intensity of the stimulus, S, grows stronger, the discharge frequency, F, increases. The relationship between S and F, known as the *intensity function*, is plotted in Fig. 7-4B for various times after the start of the stimulus (1, 2, and 3 sec). As is the case with the relationship between stimulus strength and receptor potential, here, too, for the stretch receptor, a linear relationship exists at all times during the stimulus. Since the receptor potential must attain a certain minimum magnitude (depolarization threshold of the axon; see Chapter 2) in order to trigger action potentials, a discharge starts only when the corresponding stimulus intensity, S_0, in Fig. 7-4B is exceeded. S_0 is termed the *threshold stimulus* of the receptor. The intensity functions in Fig. 7-4B are described by expressions of the form $F = k \times (S - S_0)$. The factor k is the slope of the straight line. It becomes smaller during the course of the stimulus. This is also an expression of adaptation.

Experiments have shown that for most receptors the intensity function is *nonlinear* and can be described by a relationship in the form $F = k \times (S - S_0)^n$. The exponent n is a characteristic constant for each receptor. Such an expression is called a power function. The stimulus intensity, S, reduced by the stimulus threshold S_0, is raised to the nth power. At $n < 1$ and $n > 1$ the power function has its convexity upward and downward, respectively (Fig. 7-5). For $n = 1$ we find the linear intensity function (for example, of the stretch receptor). For most of the receptors described so far, the power functions that apply have exponents n with values between 0.5 and 1.0.

To test whether an experimentally determined intensity function

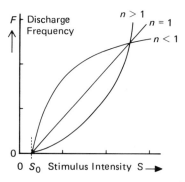

Fig. 7-5. Shape of power functions with various exponents. In the linear coordinate system the power functions have the characteristic shape as shown, depending on whether the exponent is $n < 1$, > 1, or $= 1$.

can be represented by a power function, the measured values of the stimulus intensity/discharge frequency are plotted in a double logarithmic coordinate system. Each power function becomes a straight line in such a coordinate system because logarithmic expression of the power function gives

$$\log F = \log k + n \times \log (S - S_0)$$

which is the equation for a straight line with slope n. If the plotted values in the double logarithmic coordinate system can be approximated by a straight line, then the relationship is a power function. The exponent n can be determined directly as the slope of this straight line.

Now please check what you have learned about receptors.

Q 7.1 Into which four groups can the receptors of mammals be classified according to their adequate stimulus?

Q 7.2 The receptor potential
    a. is an all-or-nothing response of a receptor cell that occurs only for stimuli above a stimulus threshold.
    b. is a depolarization of the receptive membrane whose amplitude increases as the stimulus intensity increases.
    c. spreads electrotonically to the axon membrane and acts there as a generator for propagated action potentials.
    d. is generated by an increase in conductance specifically for H^+ ions.
    e. increases slowly with constant stimulus and lasts as long as the stimulus.
    More than one answer is correct.

Q 7.3 The discharge frequency in the afferent axon of many receptors
    a. increases with increasing stimulus intensity.
    b. increases during the course of a stimulus of constant intensity.
    c. declines in the course of a stimulus of constant intensity.
    d. is zero at subthreshold stimulus strength.
    e. is not dependent on the magnitude of the receptor potential.
    More than one answer is correct.

Q 7.4 In many receptors a power function describes the
    a. time course of the adaptation.
    b. time course of the receptor potential with increasing stimulus strength.
    c. relationship between the discharge frequency, F, and the amount of stimulus intensity by which the stimulus threshold, S_0, is exceeded.
    d. relationship between the amount of increase in conductance at the receptive membrane and the magnitude of the receptor potential.

7.2   Afferent Nerves to the Spinal Cord and Their Spinal Connections; Ascending Pathways

Peripheral nerves, dorsal roots, and their innervation areas.   The nerve impulses issuing from the receptors are conducted to the CNS by the afferent axons. On the way to the CNS the nerve fibers combine in bundles to form the *peripheral nerves* (see Sec. 1-3). If a cutaneous nerve is transected as a result of an injury, then cutaneous stimuli are no longer perceived in a relatively sharply defined area. The skin region in which this sensory loss occurs is known as the *innervation area* of the transected nerve or nerve branch. The sharp delineation is due to the fact that overlapping of neighboring innervation areas of cutaneous nerves is small (Fig. 7-6A).

When a cutaneous nerve is transected, not only is one aware of the sensory loss, but it is also noticed that the skin of the affected region becomes dry and brittle. This is because the innervation of the sweat glands by the autonomic efferents, which also run in the cutaneous nerves, are likewise interrupted (see Sec. 1-3).

All afferent fibers from skin, muscles, joints, and intestinal organs enter the spinal cord by the *dorsal roots* (see Fig. 1-11). The dorsal and the ventral roots of a spinal segment combine to form the *spinal nerve*, which is thus a bundle of cutaneous, muscle, joint, and visceral nerve fibers (both afferent and efferent fibers). A particular peripheral region is represented afferently in each dorsal root. However, the region is not formed simply by the combining of innervation regions of peripheral nerves. The nerve fibers are in fact rebundled on the way to the spinal cord as shown in Fig. 7-6B for cutaneous nerves.

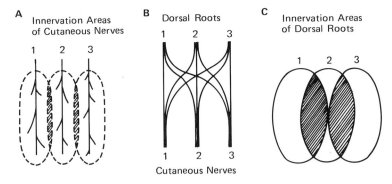

Fig. 7-6.   Innervation areas of cutaneous nerves and dorsal roots (schematic). The innervation areas of nerve branches are sharply delineated and exhibit little overlapping (A). Because of the the rebundling of peripheral nerves to spinal nerves (B) the innervation areas of dorsal roots are less sharply delineated and overlap (C).

Each peripheral nerve contains fibers emanating from several adjacent spinal nerves, and, conversely, fibers of each spinal nerve go to various peripheral nerves. As a result of this rebundling of the nerve fibers the region innervated by a spinal nerve or a dorsal root is less precisely delineated than that of a peripheral nerve. The areas innervated by neighboring spinal nerves overlap considerably (Fig. 7-6C). When a nerve is cut near the periphery we observe a sensory loss with well defined boundaries in the organ innervated by the nerve (either the skin, the muscle, the joints, or the viscera). On the other hand, cutting a dorsal root or a spinal nerve decreases the density of the innervation in all these organs.

The cutaneous area innervated by a spinal nerve is called a *dermatome*. The dermatomes are arranged at the surface of the body in the same sequence as the corresponding spinal cord segments. For example, the innervation of the pelvic region issues from spinal cord segments that are more distant from the brain than the segments that innervate the shoulder. Corresponding to this topographical relationship between areas of the body surface and the segments of the spinal cord, the latter is divided into four main sections (Fig. 7-7): cervical cord, thoracic cord, lumbar cord, and sacral cord. The approximate boundaries of the associated dermatomes are shown in Fig. 7-7.

The topographical relationship between segments of the spinal cord and certain areas of the skin, the musculature, the joints, and the viscera can be understood if one considers the embryonic development of vertebrates. The specialization of the nervous system first becomes apparent at the early embryonic stage, while the remaining

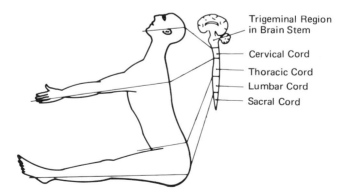

Fig. 7-7. Topographical relationship between areas of body surface and segments of the spinal cord. The lines give the approximate subdivisions of the skin surface (left) related to the four main sections of the spinal cord (right). (Diagram modified from Ruch and Patton, *Physiology and Biophysics*, Saunders, Philadelphia, 1966.)

organs are as yet not differentiated. However, at this stage it is already possible to detect the organization of the cord into segments. Each of the 31 spinal cord segments is related topographically to adjacent, still undifferentiated cells. This topographical relationship of the primitive segments remains unchanged as the embryo develops. The growth of the nerve cells is completed sooner than that of the other body tissue so that the close proximity of spinal cord segments and the associated innervated organs is usually not retained. Because of these different growth phases, the spinal cord, for example, is considerably shorter than the vertebral column. The spinal nerves of the lower half of the body therefore at first run caudally in the vertebral canal, emerging from it at the appropriate vertebral processes.

Circuitry of the afferent fibers in the spinal cord segment. The afferents entering the spinal cord through the dorsal roots divide into varying numbers of branches. These branches, called collaterals, for the most part form *synaptic contacts* with neurons that are located in the gray matter of the spinal cord. Each spinal neuron is connected with several afferent fibers, and, conversely, each afferent fiber forms synapses with several spinal neurons. Distinct functional connections are superimposed on this general principle of *convergence/ divergence,* with which we are already familiar from Chapter 4. Examples of these functional connections have been given in Chapters 4 and 6: the monosynaptic stretch reflex of the spindle afferents of a muscle, the mutual inhibition of the stretch reflexes of antagonistic muscles, and the polysynaptic reflexes of cutaneous and visceral afferents to motoneurons. These functional connections mean that the sensory impulses from the skin, the muscles, the joints, and the viscera are processed or *integrated* in a segment. The processing of the impulses at the level of a spinal segment is symbolized diagrammatically in the lower part of Fig. 7-8 by the synaptic connection of a dorsal root fiber with a motoneuron (A). The connection is monosynaptic only in the special case of the stretch reflex. We can see from examples taken from our normal daily existence that segmental integration takes place unconsciously (for example, the interplay of agonist and antagonist during walking).

The sensory function of the afferent nerves, however, is not limited to one particular spinal segment. Some of the information arriving by the dorsal root fibers also leaves the segment again via collaterals of the afferent fibers and axons of spinal cord neurons, both of which run in the white matter. As a result, connections are made with neighboring segments (propriospinal pathways), and long axons extend to the portions of the CNS located outside the spinal cord, that is, supraspinally.

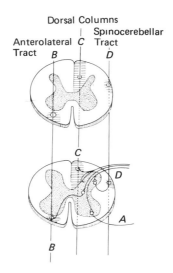

Fig. 7-8. Ascending pathways in the spinal cord. Besides the connections with motor efferents (A) at the segmental level, afferent fibers can also be connected with pathways leading to the brain. The most important of these pathways are the anterolateral tract (B), the dorsal column (C), and the spinocerebellar tract (D).

Ascending tracts in the spinal cord. The dorsal root fibers in Fig. 7-8 are connected synaptically with two neurons whose axons enter the *white* matter. One of the afferent fibers sends a collateral *directly* to the white matter. Long axons run in the three regions of the white matter which are specially indicated in Fig. 7-8. These axons transmit sensory information to the supraspinal sections of the CNS. A bundle of long axons in the spinal cord is called a *tract*, or *column*. The two synaptically relayed pathways B and D in Fig. 7-8 are called the *anterolateral* tract (B) and the *spinocerebellar* tract (D). Collaterals of the afferent fibers enter the *dorsal column* (C) directly, that is, without being relayed synaptically. Each afferent fiber can be connected with several ascending pathways and, in addition, with the motor efferents at the segmental level. This illustrates the principle of divergence. In an extreme case, one fiber can make simultaneously all the connections in Fig. 7-8.

Direct collaterals from the thick myelinated afferents of muscles, skin, joints, and viscera run in the *dorsal column* (C in Fig. 7-8). These are mainly Group I and Group II fibers (see Tables 1-1 and 1-2), which come from low threshold *mechanoreceptors* of the innervated areas in question. The function of the dorsal column is chiefly to transmit signals to the brain about tactile events on the skin and the position of the limbs. These signals are perceived consciously and the sensory abilities of the dorsal column system are termed *tactile sensitivity* and *posture sense*, respectively. The high degree of spatial resolution is a special characteristic of the perception of mechanical cutaneous stimuli via the dorsal column. This ability to differentiate spatially between tactile stimuli is particularly affected when interruptions occur in the dorsal column. For example, a person who has suffered this sort of lesion cannot, with his eyes closed, recognize an object by touching it, nor can he recognize figures traced on his skin.

These two abilities are easy to check out yourself on a test person (eyes closed) by the following tests.

    1. Recognition of various objects:

        a. through contact with the skin, for example, on upper arm.

        b. by touching with the fingers.

    2. Recognition of numbers traced with a fairly blunt object at various regions on the body surface. How big must the figures be traced at the various points in order to be recognized distinctly?

    3. Place the two points of a blunt pair of dividers simultaneously on the skin and measure the minimum distance between the points at which the test subject can recognize the stimulus as a two-point stimulus (two-point threshold). Carry out the test at various areas on the body.

The tactile sense abilities that can be checked by these tests require an intact dorsal column. Lesions of the dorsal column (for example, in the case of partial transection of the spinal cord) can be diagnosed with such tests.

The *anterolateral tract* (B in Fig. 7-8), which ascends crossed on the opposite side of the spinal cord, receives afferent impulses mainly from the *high-threshold* receptors (nociceptors) and the *thermo-receptors*. When pain cannot be controlled in any other way (for example, in the case of inoperable tumors) selective transection of the anterolateral tract (cordotomy) can bring relief to a patient. However, sensitivity to temperature also disappears when this operation is performed. The lesion affects the dermatomes of all the spinal nerves situated below (caudally from) the point of transection. When the anterolateral tract is interrupted, only the tactile stimulus, which is usually coupled with thermal and painful stimuli, is transmitted to the brain via the dorsal column. In this case, when, for example, only the tactile portion of a needle prick or of a contact with a warm object is perceived, we speak of *dissociated sensory loss*.

The *spinocerebellar* tract, whose axons have for the most part not crossed the spinal cord midline, transmits information chiefly from *mechanoreceptors* of skin, muscles, and joints to the cerebellum. The cerebellum uses these sensory inputs to regulate the coordination of muscle groups involved in a particular movement (see Chapter 6). This process of coordination is not perceived consciously. Here, just as in the case of segmental integration, we have an example of the fact that sensory information does not necessarily lead to conscious perception.

The axons arising from adjacent sections of the body retain their spatial relationships to one another within the ascending pathways. As a result, we find a *topographical order* within the pathways as shown in diagrammatic form in Fig. 7-9 for the dorsal and the anterolateral columns in the region of the cervical cord. The new axons, which join a pathway as it ascends in the spinal cord, always do so from the side of the gray matter. Given only superficial damage (tumor, injury) to the anterolateral tract in the region of the cervical vertebral column, sensory deficits should first of all be expected in the lower half of the body.

The afferent fibers of the head region, that is, the nerves of the eyes, the labyrinth, the ear, and the skin of the face as well as the gustatory nerves, enter the brain stem directly (the brain stem is the region of the CNS located between the spinal cord and the cerebrum; see Fig. 6-13). The somatic innervation of the face region, that is, of the skin of the face, the lips, parts of the tongue, and the teeth, takes place by the *trigeminus* nerve. Like the spinal cord afferents, this nerve is connected with pathways that ascend to the cerebrum.

The sensory impulses arriving via the afferent nerves are thus processed at the segmental level in the spinal cord and fed to motor efferents, and in addition they are conducted by the long ascending pathways to the brain. While the impulses are being transmitted along

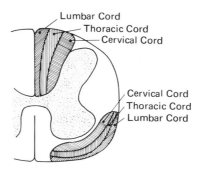

Lumbar Cord
Thoracic Cord
Cervical Cord

Cervical Cord
Thoracic Cord
Lumbar Cord

Fig. 7-9. Topographical arrangement of the ascending pathways. Diagrammatical cross section through the upper part of the cervical cord. New axons joining a pathway as it ascends in the spinal cord always do so from the side of the gray matter. This results in a topographical arrangement of the pathways corresponding to the sites of origin of the afferent fibers.

the ascending pathways, the information about the peripheral stimuli is retained. For example, an increase in the intensity of a stimulus on the skin will lead in ascending axons as well to an increase in the mean discharge frequency, fully in keeping with the conditions of the receptors. When the afferent fibers are relayed synaptically to the neurons in the gray matter, the processes we studied in Chapter 3 take effect, for example, temporal and spatial facilitation and inhibition. As a result, the ingoing trains of impulses can be modified in a wide variety of ways.

What you have learned in this section should enable you to answer the following questions.

Q 7.5 Please draw a cross section through the spinal cord showing the afferent fibers and their connections with segmental efferents and ascending pathways.

Q 7.6 Transection of a cutaneous nerve near the periphery causes
a. loss of temperature and pain sensations only.
b. dry skin in the affected innervation area as a result of denervation of the sweat glands.
c. flaccid paralysis as a result of interruption of the extrinsic reflex arc.
d. loss of input from high- and low-threshold mechanoreceptors and thermoreceptors.
More than one answer is correct.

Q 7.7 Which nerve fibers are interrupted when a dorsal root is destroyed?
a. The efferent motor and sympathetic fibers.
b. The afferent fibers from skin, muscles, joints, and viscera.
c. Only the afferent fibers from the skin.
Which fibers are interrupted when a spinal nerve is destroyed?
d. Only the afferent fibers
e. All afferent and efferent fibers of the corresponding half of the segment.

Q 7.8 As a result of a transverse lesion, the left half of the thoracic cord is completely severed. Which of the following symptoms are observed? (More than one answer is correct)
a. Paralysis of the left leg as a result of interruption of the pyramidal pathway.
b. Temperature and pain sensations extinguished on the left side of the body.
c. Temperature and pain sensations extinguished in the right buttock.
d. Figures traced on the dorsum of the right foot can be recognized.
e. Light touching of the left leg cannot be localized exactly.

7.3 The Thalamocortical Projection of the Sensory Periphery

The thalamus as a central afferent relay. So far, we have studied the processing of sensory impulses in the spinal cord and the parts of the brain that play an important role in motor control. These functions of the CNS take place to a large extent unconsciously. We will now concentrate on those functions of the CNS that can result in *conscious perception* of stimuli. To do this, taking the somatosensory system as an example, we must trace the course of the sensory pathways, that is, the dorsal column and the anterolateral tract, issuing from the spinal cord.

First, Fig. 7-10 gives a general view of the anatomy of the supraspinal parts of the brain. The spinal cord connects with the *medulla oblongata,* adjacent to which lies the *pons,* followed by the *mesencephalon.* These three parts together are usually termed the *brain stem.* The *cerebellum* appears as a dorsal appendix of the brain stem. We have already seen that parts of the brain stem as well as of the

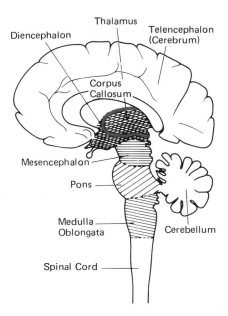

Fig. 7-10. Macroscopic division of the CNS. The seven different regions into which the CNS is divided are labeled. The medulla oblongata, the pons, and the midbrain together are known as the brain stem. The thalamus (red marking), which is of particular importance for the sensory system, is part of the diencephalon.

cerebellum are important components of the motor system (see Chapter 6). The greatest part of the brain is the *telencephalon*, or the *cerebrum*, which consists of two largely separate halves, the two *hemispheres*. The two halves of the cerebrum are connected with one another by nerve fiber fasciculi which run chiefly in the *corpus callosum* (perpendicular to the plane of the diagram in Fig. 7-10). The region between the brain stem and the cerebrum is called the *diencephalon*. The region of the diencephalon, marked off in red, contains an accumulation of ganglia which are of great importance for the sensory systems. This part of the diencephalon is called the *thalamus* and, with the exception of the olfactory nerve, activity reaches it from all sensory systems.

A knowledge of the names and the locations of the individual subdivisions of the brain is essential if you are to follow what comes next. You should now be in a position to draw a sketch of the CNS showing the subdivisions and naming the parts.

The afferents from the trunk are connected with the thalamus by the dorsal column and the anterolateral tract (Fig. 7-11). As we have learned, the dorsal column consists of collaterals from the peripheral nerve fibers. These are synaptically relayed in the *dorsal column nuclei* of the medulla oblongata. The postsynaptic axons cross to the opposite (that is, contralateral) side and then run parallel to the fibers

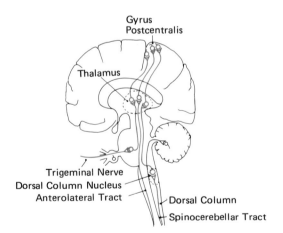

Fig. 7-11. Connection of the ascending pathways in the brain. The spinocerebellar tract transmits the afferent activity from the spinal cord to the cerebellum. The anterolateral tract and the dorsal columns (after being relayed synaptically in the dorsal column nuclei) conduct the afferent activity to the thalamus. The afferents from the face region enter the brain stem via the trigeminal nerve and also run to the thalamus. The thalamic neurons project onto the sensory cortex.

of the anterolateral tract through the brain stem to the thalamus. The trigeminal nerve, which contains the somatic afferents of the face region, is also relayed in the pons (Fig. 7-11) to a pathway that likewise crosses the midline of the brain stem and runs to the thalamus. You now know the three pathways by which the somatic and the visceral afferents reach the thalamus. These pathways form synaptic connections with neurons which are situated in circumscribed parts of the thalamus, the *specific relay nuclei* of the somatosensory system. Nuclei are termed specific when they receive their afferent input selectively from a certain sensory organ. Since the three named afferent pathways cross to the opposite side in the spinal cord or in the brain stem, the specific nuclei of the left half of the thalamus are connected with the periphery of the right side of the body, and vice versa.

An experiment demonstrating some properites of specific somatosensory thalamic neurons is shown in Fig. 7-12. Part A of the figure shows a frontal section through the brain as viewed from the rear. A microelectrode to record the impulse activity of individual cells is inserted from above into the right half of the thalamus (marked in red). The crosshatched area indicates approximately the position of the specific nucleus for the somatosensory system of the trunk, and it is

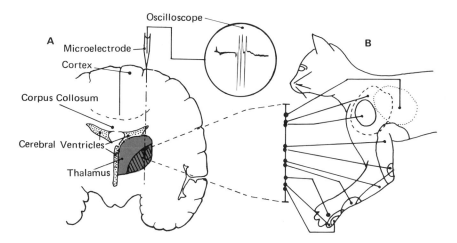

Fig. 7-12. Projection of the body surface onto individual thalamus neurons. A: Using a microelectrode inserted through the cerebrum into certain regions of the thalamus, it is possible to record action potentials of individual thalamus neurons. B: All the neurons recorded along one electrode track which were activated by mechanical stimuli in the associated regions of the body surface (receptive fields of the neurons). (From V.B. Mountcastle, *Medical Physiology*, Vol. II, Mosby, St. Louis, 1968.)

here that the anterolateral tract and the projection of the dorsal column terminate. In this region the microelectrode records from neurons that can be activated by mechanical stimuli of the skin. This is demonstrated by the action potentials on the oscilloscope screen in Fig. 7-12*A*.

The track of the microelectrode through the thalamic nucleus is shown on an expanded scale in Fig. 7-12*B*. Each point along the track indicates the position of a neuron from which recordings could be made. The most important results of this experiment are as follows.

1.   Each neuron could be activated only by applying mechanical stimuli to the relevant area encircled in the left front leg of the animal (cat). This area is the receptive field of the neuron. Each thalamic neuron is generally activated by several adjacent peripheral receptors (convergence). These adjacent receptors form the receptive field of the thalamic neuron.

2.   It will be noticed in Fig. 7-12*B* that on the average receptive fields become smaller as they are located further along the extremity toward the toe. The thalamic neurons that are assigned to the forepaw, and in man to the hand, thus have small receptive fields. As a result, a good spatial resolution is achieved in the projection of the hand onto the thalamus. This observation is probably a neurophysiological correlate of the excellent spatial discriminative ability of the human hand. (You should test this by recognizing differences in the surface roughness of objects by tactile exploration with your fingers; compare with the visual discrimination of the same surfaces!)

3.   Adjacent body regions project onto adjacent regions in the specific thalamic nucleus. There is thus a *somatotopic* organization. This topographical relationship of the periphery to the CNS is already present in the ascending pathways (see Fig. 7-9).

The regions of the thalamus that are not crosshatched in Fig. 7-12*A* are partly filled with ganglia onto which the afferents from other sensory organs project (for example, eye, inner ear). Therefore, these are the specific nuclei of these particular sensory systems. The specific nuclei, which are excited by one sensory organ only, are always characterized by a topographically organized projection of the sensory surface, this being generally termed somatotopic organization. Apart from these specific thalamic nuclei, we also find regions with neurons onto which afferents from several different sense organs converge (for example, eye + vestibular organ + skin). These so-called *nonspecific nuclei* lack any topographical relationship to the periphery. A further characteristic of nonspecific nuclei is that they are activated from the periphery after latencies much longer than those for the specific nuclei. From this it may be concluded that they are reached via neuronal pathways that contain considerably more synapses than the pathways to the specific nuclei. In Sec. 7.4 you will learn something about the functional importance of the nonspecific thalamic nuclei.

Afferents from all the sense organs (with the exception of the olfactory organ) are thus relayed in the specific nuclei of the thalamus. Efferent axons from these nuclei run to certain regions of the cerebral cortex. Accordingly, the thalamus can be regarded as a central synaptic relay for all the afferent systems on the way to the cortex.

The primary sensory projection to the cortex. The neurons in the specific thalamic nucleus for the body surface send out axons to the *Gyrus postcentralis* (Fig. 7-11) on the same side of the brain. This region of the cortex is situated directly behind the central sulcus (Sulcus centralis), which runs as a deep groove transversely over the cerebrum. The cortical region of the Gyrus postcentralis is called the *sensory cortex* of the body periphery or, synonymously, the *somatosensory cortex* (Fig. 7-13).

Similarly, afferents from the eye and the ear—after being relayed in the relevant specific thalamic nuclei—run to certain cortical regions whose positions are shown in Fig. 7-13. These regions are called the sensory cortex of the eye or the ear (visual or auditory cortex).

A strict topographical order, called the *somatotopic projection,* exists between the periphery of the body and the somatosensory cortex on the opposite side. You have already come across a similar topographical order in the thalamus. In Fig. 7-13 this somatotopic

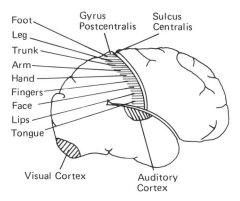

Fig. 7-13. Primary sensory projection of the body onto the cortex. The various regions of the body are connected with specific areas on the Gyrus postcentralis as labeled. This is known as somatotopic projection. The corresponding primary projection regions of eye and inner ear are also shown.

projection of the periphery of the body is indicated by corresponding labeling. This topographical order is quite similar to the way in which the motor cortex is related to the musculature of the body periphery (see Fig. 6-9). It is indicated in Fig. 7-13 that the hand and the face have cortical projection areas that in each case are about as large as the projection fields of trunk and leg together. It is a general law that organs with a particularly high receptor density (for example, fingers, lips) project onto correspondingly large neuron populations in the somatosensory cortex. This feature is also a correlate of the high discriminatory capability of such sensory surfaces, as already discussed in the section on the thalamus.

In animal experiments the somatotopic organization, that is, the orderly projection of the body periphery onto the sensory cortex, is studied by recording *evoked potentials,* as shown in Fig. 7-14A. The anesthetized animal is stimulated, for example, by individual electric shocks at the periphery. The potentials evoked in the cortex are recorded with an electrode that is positioned in various places. When a point at the periphery is stimulated, evoked potentials can be recorded in the cortex; the time course of such a potential is shown in Fig. 7-14B. The type of potential recorded is one to which the extracellular currents of many neurons in the vicinity of the electrode contribute; it is called a *mass potential.*

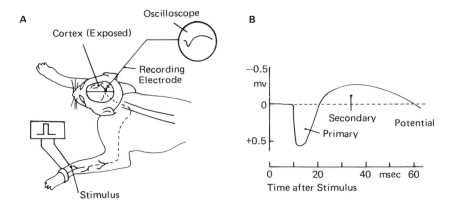

Fig. 7-14. Measuring evoked potentials in the cortex (diagrammatic view). *A:* Evoked potentials can be recorded in the exposed cortex when peripheral stimuli are applied. The characteristic time course of these potentials is shown in *B.* The (positive) primary potential can be recorded only from the primary sensory projection area in the case of a circumscribed peripheral stimulus, while a secondary potential is generated over large areas of the cortex. (Modified from P. Glees, in Landois-Rosemann, *Lehrbuch der Physiologie des Menschen*, Urban & Schwarzenberg, Munich, 1962.)

After the stimulus, an initial change in potential occurs with a latent period of 10 msec, and it reaches its maximum value quickly. This early response is called a *primary* evoked potential. It is only found in a strictly circumscribed region of the cortex, namely, the *cortical projection field* of the peripheral point.

The late response that follows after the primary evoked potential shown in Fig. 7-14B lasts about 50 msec (in the example used in Fig. 7-14) and is called the *secondary* evoked potential. This potential is found in a more extensive region of the cortex, its time course showing a wide variation.

The primary responses originate from neurons on which the axons from the specific nuclei of the thalamus end (see Fig. 7-11). The most direct sensory connection between periphery and cortex runs along these paths. The relatively long latent period of the secondary response indicates that it is generated only after the activity has passed through additional synapses. The nonspecific thalamic nuclei are also involved here.

By stimulating systematically the entire periphery point by point and recording the corresponding activity in the cortex, "maps" of the sensory cortical projections have been drawn up, as shown in Fig. 7-13. A corresponding efferent map of the motor cortex and the muscles assigned to it has already been given in Chapter 6.

By measuring the cortical mass potentials the primary projection areas of other sense organs can be determined as well. The receptors in the retina of the eye project into a circumscribed region in the occipital lobe of the brain; the receptors of the inner ear project onto the temporal lobes (see Fig. 7-13). Here, too, a somatotopic relationship exists between the peripheral sensory surface and the cortex.

With the technique described in Fig. 7-14 potential changes are recorded that are made up of the extracellular currents of a very large number of neurons. Using microelectrodes individual neurons are found in the primary sensory areas that respond to peripheral stimulation with action potentials after a short latent period. Such cells are very frequently activated by stimulation of a *particular* type of receptor. For example, in the somatosensory cortex of the monkey two types of neurons could be identified, each of which responded to either one of two well-known types of cutaneous mechanoreceptors.

The cortex consists of a layer of neurons several millimeters thick. The cortical cells activated from a certain receptive field in the periphery are arranged in a column perpendicular to the surface of the cortex (columnar organization). It must be assumed that the processing of the incoming volleys in such a neuronal unit is very complex. The information is transmitted in this processed form to other cortical regions, for example, to the motor cortex on the Gyrus praecentralis or to the so-called association areas. Our knowledge of the interaction of such collective groups of neurons is still extremely limited. Above all, we still have no idea how the neuronal events (for example, changes in potential) give rise to what we call conscious perception.

The thalamocortical system and conscious sensory perception; other cortical regions. In the following we will discuss two experiments indicating that the sensory cortex plays an important role in conscious sensory perception and highly developed discriminatory sensory performance. Let us take the case of a conscious patient whose cortex has been partially exposed (using local anesthesia) for therapeutic reasons. If the sensory cortex is stimulated with a fine electrode then the patient reports sensations in *circumscribed* areas of the body periphery. When, for example, the hand region in the somatosensory cortex is stimulated, the patient perceives tactile stimuli on his hand. Stimulation in the visual cortex generates the sensation of flashes of light. By direct stimulation of the sensory cortex, conscious sensations can therefore be triggered *without* activation of the afferent pathways via the peripheral nerves, the spinal cord, and the specific nuclei of the thalamus. However, stimulation of the cortex never produces sensations of pain.

In monkeys the experimental removal of circumscribed areas of the sensory cortex causes sensory deficits in the associated peripheral areas. For example, before the operation the animals had learned to distinguish a cube from a sphere by touch alone. After removal of the sensory cortical hand region this *discriminatory* ability was lost and could not be relearned. Similar findings also have been reported in humans suffering from circumscribed damage to the sensory cortex (for example, bullet wounds, tumors). However, pain is experienced just as before; it is only the ability to pinpoint exactly the source of the pain that is disturbed.

From the results of local stimulation of the cortex and removal of parts of the cortex it can therefore be concluded that the sensory cortex is somatotopically organized in man too, and the sensory cortex is involved in conscious sensory perception.

The primary sensory projection areas of the cortex together with the motor cortex mentioned earlier (see Chapter 6) account for about 20 percent of the cortical area. The remaining area of the cortex is much larger, but all that can be recorded here with a surface electrode are the secondary evoked potentials (Fig. 7-14B). These large areas of the cortex in which secondary evoked potentials are recorded when a sense organ is stimulated usually overlap to a considerable extent.

Thus the greater part of the cortical area is *not* associated electrophysiologically with one particular sense organ.

The function of these cortical regions can be assessed from the sensory loss that occurrs when circumscribed damage is suffered. For example, if a certain region in the vicinity of the visual cortex is injured, then symptoms occur that are referred to as *visual agnosia*. A patient with the clinical symptoms of visual agnosia retains his power of sight fully intact and can, for example, avoid obstacles or reach for objects. However, he often cannot *recognize* what the objects actually are. If a person with this type of lesion looks at a sponge, for instance, he cannot identify it when asked to do so. But if he handles the sponge, then he recognizes it by his tactile sense.

The regions to which such higher sensory functions can be assigned on the basis of lesion symptoms are called the association areas of the cortex. In primates, and in particular in man, they are much more extensive than in other mammals. A specific human association area is linked with the recognition and the articulation of speech sounds ("speech center"). Very little neurophysiological research has been done so far on association areas.

Answer the following questions to check the knowledge you have acquired.

Q 7.9   Somatotopic projection means that the (more than one answer is correct)
    a. soma of the nerve cell puts out branches in certain directions.
    b. peripheral sensory surface has a "point-to-point" topographical relationship with the sensory cortex.
    c. peripheral regions project on the sensory cortex.
    d. cells of the sensory cortex are related geometrically to those of the motor cortex.

Q 7.10   The neurons of the specific nuclei of the thalamus obtain their afferent input from
    a. one sensory organ via at least seven synapses.
    b. several sense organs simultaneously via at least three synapses.
    c. the thermal and the pain afferents of the skin via the cerebellum.
    d. one sensory organ via at least two synapses.

Q 7.11   Which of the following statements apply when the arm and the hand regions of the right somatosensory cortex are removed? (More than one answer is correct.)
    a. Objects cannot be distinguished by touching with the right hand.
    b. The voluntary motor control of the left arm is unaffected

because the motor cortex receives the necessary afferents via
the cerebellum.

c. Pain stimulation of the left hand is perceived but it cannot
be exactly localized.

d. No pain is felt in the left hand.

7.4   Electroencephalogram (EEG) and the Conscious State

Definition, origin, and recording of the EEG.   In the preceding
section we learned that evoked potentials can be recorded from the
cortex during peripheral stimulation. These evoked potentials were
interpreted as the sum of the extracellular currents of synchronously
activated cortical neurons. But, even *without* peripheral stimulation,
apparently spontaneous fluctuations in potential can be recorded from
all regions of the cerebral cortex. This recording is known as an
electroencephalogram, or *EEG*. Typical examples of EEGs are shown
in Fig. 7-15. These were, in fact, recorded from the intact skull. The
ability to record the EEG in the intact human head is of great practical
significance for both experimental neurophysiology and clinical diagnostic work. It is possible to record the EEG through the skull be-

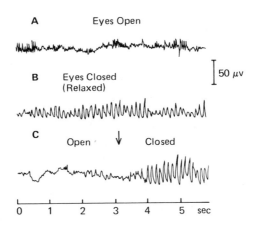

Fig. 7-15.   Examples of various types of electroencephalograms (EEGs).
The EEGs recorded on the head of an awake person consist of many small
irregular fluctuations in potential per unit time when the subject is alert (*A*);
while in the relaxed state (eyes closed, *B*) the fluctuations have a pronounced
periodicity (α rhythm). The transition to the relaxed state is shown in *C*.

cause the latter is not an electric insulator. In this case, the recording electrodes are relatively far removed from the sources of the EEG currents in the cortex, and this is why the amplitude of the recorded potentials is small. If the EEG is recorded directly at the surface of the cortex, then it is larger than the measurements taken through the intact skull by a factor of approximately 10. Recording of the EEG through the skull has its parallel in the recording of the cardiac action currents through the intact chest wall (electrocardiogram, or ECG).

The EEGs in Fig. 7-15*A* and *B* were recorded in immediate succession at the back of the head of an awake person. In *A* the eyes were open. In *B* they were closed. In Fig. 7-15, where the subject had his eyes closed, a pronounced rhythm is detectable in the potential fluctuations: the EEG is *synchronized*. In contrast, the EEG in Fig. 7-15*A* is *desynchronized*. The rhythm of the synchronized EEG in Fig. 7-15*B* consists mainly of periodical fluctuations in potential, averaging about 8 to 10 per second. This periodicity, which occurs particularly in the relaxed state with the eyes closed (that is, with visual stimuli eliminated), is called the α rhythm. In the desynchronized EEG higher frequencies prevail (up to 30 per second); this type of periodicity is called the β rhythm. Fig. 7-15*C* shows how the desynchronized EEG converts to the synchronized state when the eyes are closed.

A comparison of the EEGs with *intracellular* measurements from cortical cells has shown that the fluctuations in potential at the surface of the cortex are chiefly caused by the extracellular currents that flow when cortical cells are synaptically activated. As already stated in the section on cortical projection fields, a large-area electrode records the composite of the extracellular currents of all the neurons in the vicinity of the electrode. If recordings are taken directly from the surface of the cortex with an electrode having a surface of, say, 1 mm^2, then somewhere in the order of 100,000 neurons will be located beneath the electrode in a range down to a depth of 0.5 mm. When the recording is made through the skull it can be estimated that the area contributing to the electrode is larger by a factor of at least 10. The electrode thus records the total activity of about 10^6 nerve cells. Large-amplitude fluctuations in the mass potentials can only occur when a major fraction of the neurons beneath the electrode are synaptically activated at the same time (synchronously). Cells with an elongated dendritic tree theoretically can make particularly large contributions to the compound potential at the cortical surface. It must be assumed therefore that the current sources for the EEG are represented primarily by parallel-arranged dendritic structures of fairly deeply located neurons that extend to the surface of the cortex.

The EEG in various sleeping and waking states.   Research has shown that the EEG can be used as an indicator of various states of normal and abnormal brain activity. Characteristic potential patterns occur, depending on the level of consciousness of the test person and on certain pathological changes of the CNS. We have already come across an example of the first instance in Fig. 7-15: relaxation with elimination of external stimuli (eyes closed) is coupled with a synchronized EEG (α rhythm).

Strong synchronization also occurs in deep sleep (Fig. 7-16C). The predominant frequency here is less than 4 per second, and it is called the δ *rhythm*. In Fig. 7-16 the deep-sleep EEG (C) is compared with the normal awake EEG (A) and the EEG of relaxed wakefulness (B, eyes closed). It will be noted that the amplitudes of the potentials become greater as the prevailing frequency becomes lower (note that the amplitude calibration scale in C is different from that in A and B). However, during sleep, the deep-sleep EEG with the slow δ rhythm does not occur all the time. Instead, this EEG alternates with phases in which the EEG is desynchronized and thus is similar to the EEG of the normal awake state. This sleep phase is therefore termed *paradoxical-sleep*. During the paradoxical-sleep phases with their desynchronized EEG, typical changes occur in certain of the sleeping person's physiological parameters. For example, heart and breathing rates are accelerated, and a particularly striking characteristic is the occurrence of *rapid eye movements*. For this reason these phases of sleep are also commonly referred to as REM

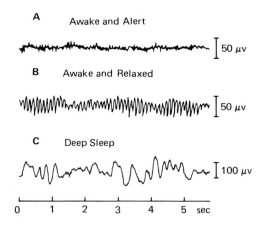

Fig. 7-16.   EEGs in the waking and deep-sleep states. A deep-sleep EEG (C) is compared with waking EEGs (A, B). Note that the potential calibration scale for C is different from that for A and B.

sleep (REM = Rapid Eye Movements). If a test person is awakened from paradoxical or REM sleep, he will report that he has just been dreaming. Paradoxical sleep with its desynchronized EEG thus characterizes *dream phases*. Deep sleep with its synchronized EEG is free from dreams.

Paradoxical, or REM, sleep occurs in all mammals. It is concluded from this that animals also dream. Normally the REM periods take up about 20 percent of the total sleeping time. If a person is prevented over a long period of time from getting paradoxical sleep, namely, by awakening him each time an EEG desynchronization starts, then behavioral changes occur (anxiety, uncertainty, increased irritability). These phenomena disappear again as soon as an undisturbed sleep sequence is permitted. However, when the return to a normal sleep pattern is made, the REM portion of the sleep is increased for several nights.

It is *empirically* confirmed that the form of the EEG and the level of consciousness are correlated. The neurophysiological knowledge of events that lead to the typical EEG characteristics and to the parallel behavioral patterns is still very incomplete. However, tests involving destruction or electrical stimulation of certain regions of the brain have shown that links with the brain stem play an important role. More details will be given in the next section.

Control of the level of consciousness by brain stem systems. We know already that the primary projection area in the sensory cortex must be intact for peripheral stimulation to be *consciously* perceived. The afferent pathways lead to the projection area via the relevant *specific* thalamic nuclei. During sleep and under anesthesia the primary evoked potential (Fig. 7-14) produced by peripheral stimulation remains unchanged, although in these cases there is obviously no *conscious perception*. We must therefore conclude that undisturbed transmission by the specific thalamic nuclei to the sensory cortex is *not in itself sufficient* to guarantee conscious sensory perception. Under anesthesia and during sleep, however, the so-called *nonspecific* system is severely suppressed (Fig. 7-17). In this system afferent activity from *all* the sense organs passes along the brain stem and the nonspecific thalamic nuclei right up to the cortex. It is characteristic for this system that inputs from different sense organs converge on the same neurons—hence the designation nonspecific system and nuclei. Another characteristic of this nonspecific system is that multisynaptic pathways are involved. On the other hand, the specific conduction by way of the thalamic relay nuclei leads via only three synapses to the cortex.

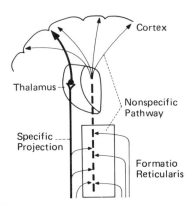

Fig. 7-17. Specific and nonspecific systems leading to the cortex (diagrammatic view). Apart from the afferent system leading to the primary projection areas by a total of three synaptic relays (specific system, see also Fig. 7-11), there are also nonspecific systems leading via the Formatio reticularis of the brain stem. They are generally multisynaptic, exhibit convergence from several sense organs, and are not somatotopically arranged.

The regions of the brain stem in which this multisynaptic conduction and nonspecific convergence from various sense organs take place are all grouped together under the single term *Formatio reticularis*, or *reticular system*. The Formatio reticularis includes all sections of the brain stem (that is, of the medulla oblongata, pons, mesencephalon) that do not possess clearly identifiable sensory or motor functions. The Formatio reticularis does not include, for example, the sensory and the motor nuclei of the cranial nerves (for example, sensory nuclei of trigeminal nerve and auditory nerve, motor nuclei for face musculature); also not included are the nuclei of the extrapyramidal motor system (Nucleus ruber, Nucleus niger). The Formatio reticularis is *not*, however, a functionally homogeneous unit. There is already much evidence to indicate that this structure can be subdivided neurophysiologically and anatomically. At the moment, the term Formatio reticularis seems to be comparable in significance with the blank areas on old maps of the world to denote still unexplored regions.

When measurement of the cortical evoked potentials was discussed a description was given of the *secondary potential* that can also be recorded outside the projection areas with a long latent period. This secondary evoked potential is brought about by *nonspecific conduction* through the Formatio reticularis and the nonspecific thalamic nuclei (Fig. 7-17). Experiments involving local electrical stimulation of the brain stem and the thalamus have shown that the synchronization of the EEG, that is, the occurrence, for example, of α and δ

rhythms, is largely determined by the nonspecific thalamic nuclei and the Formatio reticularis. At the same time, the described changes in the level of consciousness also occur. After experimental lesion of a certain part of the Formatio reticularis, the animal remains permanently unconscious, and the EEG is strongly synchronized (as in deep sleep, see Fig. 7-16C). The same thing happens in man when parts of the Formatio reticularis are destroyed, say, by tumors. From all the above results the theory has been developed that there is a constant "activating" afferent flow from the reticular system to the cerebrum that controls the state of consciousness. Therefore, the term "reticular activating system" is used to denote this functional property of the Formatio reticularis and the nonspecific thalamus. As soon as this activating afferent flow ceases, sleep or a sleeplike state sets in (anesthesia, loss of consciousness as a result of pathological processes). At the same time the EEG is synchronized.

Clinical significance of the EEG.   The EEG is gaining increasing importance as a tool for monitoring the *depth of anesthesia.* The various stages of anesthesia can be recognized from their various characteristic EEG patterns. By regulating the administration of the anesthetic it is possible to maintain a certain depth of anesthesia. *Pathological* processes in the brain can also have an effect on the EEG, a fact of considerable diagnostic importance. The following examples will illustrate these points.

For systematic recording of the EEG a large number of electrodes are distributed over the skull (Fig. 7-18A). The potential difference is recorded either between two adjacent electrodes or between each electrode and an indifferent electrode (ear). If a reduced EEG amplitude should be recorded anywhere, then this may be caused by a hematoma (hemorrhage) between cortex and skull. The hemorrhage forces the cortex downward away from the skull, and the increased distance between the current sources and the electrodes results in a reduced EEG amplitude.

Figure 7-18D shows an EEG recorded during an epileptic seizure as compared to the EEG recorded in the normal (B) and the relaxed (C) waking state. The great amplitude and the regularity in D indicate a very strong synchronization of the cortical neurons at a frequency of about 3 per second. As a result, the motor pathways emanating from the cortex are probably all rhythmically stimulated at the same time, and this leads to the powerful muscular convulsions associated with such seizures.

If the supply of oxygen to the CNS breaks down or is inadequate for a period of more than 8 to 12 min (for example, as a result of

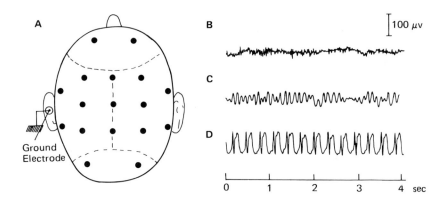

Fig. 7-18. Electrode arrangement for clinical EEG diagnosis; pathological EEG. Usually many electrodes are distributed over the skull (*A*) to record EEGs for clinical diagnostic purposes. In this way, EEGs can be recorded simultaneously from several points using a multichannel recorder (the potential is measured either between two adjacent electrodes or between each electrode and the ear electrode, the ground electrode). *D* shows an EEG recorded during an epileptic seizure. For the sake of comparison, the two basic types of waking-state EEGs (*B*, *C*) are also shown.

circulatory debility or collapse), then the CNS can suffer irreversible functional damage. In this case the EEG also fades away (isoelectric or zero-line EEG). Cessation of electrical brain activity as determined by the EEG is nowadays taken as a decisive *criterion of death*. In cases of doubt, this new definition of death has replaced the old one, which rested mainly on the cessation of circulation. It is frequently possible to revive the heart and thus the circulation even after they have been stopped for a relatively long time. But, if the CNS has been without its oxygen supply for more than about 10 min, it can no longer be revived. Once the brain is dead it is pointless to keep a person functioning by means of artificial respiration and feeding, unless organs are to be taken from the body for transplantation purposes, a practice which is at present under discussion.

Please check what you have learned. In all three questions more than one answer is correct.

Q 7.12 An EEG can be measured
    a. only in the primary sensory projection areas.
    b. in the motor cortex.
    c. in all areas of the cortex.
    d. only from the association areas.

Q 7.13 The predominant frequency of the potential changes in the EEG depends on the
    a. mental activity of the individual.

b. level of consciousness (asleep, awake).

c. degree of synchronization of cortical cells.

d. type of eye movement.

Q 7.14 The EEG is influenced mainly by a scantily studied region of the brain stem called the Formatio reticularis. It is characteristic of cells in this region that

a. afferents from various sense organs converge on them.

b. they are usually connected in multisynaptic neuronal pathways from the periphery to the cerebrum.

c. they can be activated specifically by a particular type of receptor.

7.5 The Sensory System Seen as a Communications Network

It is the role of nerve fibers to transmit signals in the form of action potentials inside the body. If the starting point of these signals is seen as a source of information and if their destination is seen as a receiver, then the nerve fiber might be compared with a telephone cable along which information is carried. This transmission of information in the nervous system can be described in terms of telecommunications engineering. This makes quantitative statements possible: the information content of a neural message can be measured, and the efficiency of neural elements in converting and transmitting information can be determined.

Encoding of information in the receptor; quantification of the information content. We already know that stimuli always have physically measurable parameters (for example, intensity of pressure on the skin, site of the stimulus on the peripheral sensory surfaces, wavelength of light and sound stimuli). These stimulus parameters constitute information concerning the body's environment. In Sec. 7.1, taking the example of the stretch receptor, it was shown how stimulus parameters determine the response of the receptors: the discharge rate in the afferent fiber (see Figs. 7-4 and 7-5) changes in the same direction as the stimulus intensity. In this case the piece of news or *information* identified as "stimulus intensity" is thus converted into the information "frequency of the action potentials." The process of converting the information is called *encoding*. This term denotes, in quite general terms, the unambiguous association of two sets of symbols (for example, the association of the alphabet with Morse signals). Thus, in each receptor a parameter of the adequate stimulus of the receptor is encoded into a sequence of neural impulses. The frequency of the action potentials is a universal information carrier for the properties of quite different stimuli, depending on the receptor in question, namely, the encoder. The significance of the sequence of action potentials in a nerve fiber is "recognized" during *decoding* in the CNS. The afferent fibers are, in fact, each connected with certain neurons (for example, Ia afferents end on homonymous motoneurons, thermoafferents end on neurons in the hypothalamus that are responsible for maintaining constant body temperature).

The quantitative determination of the *information content* of a neural message is closely connected with the number of states that can be distinguished after encoding. The following example of encoding of the stimulus intensity will show what is meant by this statement. It is known from Fig. 7.1 that the number of nerve impulses generated, for example, in a stretch receptor by a stimulus of a certain duration increases with the intensity of the stimulus. If a nerve fiber responds with only zero impulses or one impulse when the receptor is stimulated, then the receptor can provide information on two levels of stimulus intensity: stimulus strength below threshold causes no action potential, and stimulus strength above threshold causes one action potential. If the possible number of nerve impulses is zero, one, or two, then the fiber can distinguish between three levels. If a stimulus triggers a maximum of N impulses in the afferent fiber then the receptor can theoretically report $N + 1$ different levels of intensity to the CNS. This situation is illustrated by Fig. 7-19. The number of discharges, N, in the afferent fiber (ordinate) can only adopt integers.

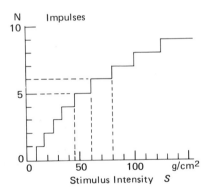

Fig. 7-19. Encoding of stimulus strength into nerve impulses. For a stimulus of a given duration only integral numbers, N, of action potentials are generated in the receptor (ordinate). The characteristic curve for coding when the stimulus intensity is varied (abscissa) is seen on closer inspection to be a discontinuous function. As a result, the accuracy with which the receptor can measure the stimulus intensity is limited. Only $N + 1$ states can be distinguished (N = maximum number of impulses per stimulus).

Consequently, the relationship with the stimulus intensity, S, (abscissa) is a discontinuous curve.

In the case of a receptor that discharges at a constant frequency in response to a long-lasting stimulus, the number of impulses, N, is the product of discharge frequency, F, and observation time, t, that is $N = F \times t$. The number of *distinguishable levels of stimulus intensity* in the afferent nerve fiber of this receptor can thus be expressed as $N + 1 = F \times t + 1$. From this relationship it follows theoretically that the number of *distinguishable levels* of stimulus intensity increases with both the *maximum frequency* to which the afferent fiber can be excited by the receptor and the duration of *observation time*, t. An upper limit for the frequency is given by the refractory period of the nerve fiber (see Chapter 2).

The unit of information in communications engineering. The quantitative unit of information in communications engineering is the *logarithm* of the number of distinguishable states of an information source. For practical reasons the logarithm to *base* 2 ($\log_2$) is selected. The reasons for this *definition* of the information unit will be outlined in the following remarks. To transmit information a set of *symbols* is needed (for example, the 26 letters of the alphabet or the digits 0 to 9) from which the source of information can make the appropriate selection. In the simplest case only two symbols, *binary symbols* (for example, 0 and 1), are used. With these the information source can report on a decision between two alternatives (for example, yes-no). From the technical standpoint binary symbols are very easy to implement (for example, bright-dark, switch positions on-off, hole-no hole on a punched tape). This is one of the reasons why this simplest of all possibilities has been adopted as the basis of the information unit.

The elementary amount of information that can be transmitted by a single binary symbol is called a *bit*. This is a very small amount of information. If long messages are to be transmitted by binary symbols, several symbols have to be strung together; in effect, one has to make *words* with the binary symbols (the "alphabet" available to form the words consists of the "letters" 0 and 1). The length of the word, that is, the number of binary symbols used per word, directly expresses the amount of information in bits. A word made up of two symbols can transmit two bits, a word of three symbols can transmit three bits, and so on. The number of words that can be formed from two binary symbols is $2^2 = 4$, namely, 00, 01, 10, 11. With three symbols $2^3 = 8$ combinations are possible, namely, 000, 001, 010, 011, 100, 101, 110, 111. With m binary digits there are obviously $n = 2^m$ possible combinations, and we can thus form $n = 2^m$ different messages, each containing m bits of information.

This definition of the information content can also be applied to cases where any other type of symbol is used as the information carrier. Any other set of symbols can, in fact, be expressed in binary digits. In order to correlate clearly a set of n symbols with binary words it is necessary for the latter to have a length averaging $m = \log_2 n$ binary digits. The reader can understand this by trying to encode the written alphabet into binary words of equal length. The necessary length of the binary words for each letter is the next integral number above $\log_2 26$, namely, 5. However, if any symbol can be replaced by a binary word, one can also say that it has the same information content (in bits) as the associated binary word. The average information content, I, of one of a set of n symbols is thus $I = \log_2 n$.

The foregoing statements also apply to the encoding process in the receptor. Here the set of symbols is the number of distinguishable states of the discharge response in the afferent nerve, which we determined above to be $n = F_{max} \times t + 1$. The information content relating to the stimulus intensity in the example given in Fig. 7-19 is thus $I = \log_2(F_{max} \times t + 1)$. This relationship between the maximal discharge frequency, F_{max}, the observation time, t, and the information content, I, is shown in Fig. 7-20. The various curves are plotted for different observation times, t. The observation period t obviously plays a decisive role in determining the number of bits transmitted. The CNS requires a certain amount of time to receive information from the receptors through a sequence of afferent impulses. If we experimentally reduce the duration of a pressure stimulus in stages,

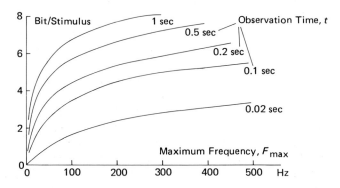

Fig. 7-20. Information capacity of a nerve fiber. The information content, I, in bits per stimulus (ordinate) is plotted as a function of the maximum discharge frequency, F_{max}, of a nerve fiber (abscissa) according to the relationship $I = \log_2 (F_{max} \times t + 1)$. The parameter of the family of curves is the observation time, t.

then the CNS receives less and less information on the intensity of the stimulus.

The intensity of the stimulus is thus one of the stimulus parameters whose information content is measurable quantitatively after encoding in the receptor. Apart from the intensity, stimuli usually have other characteristics that are relevant to the organism and must therefore be reported. The information on the spatial extent of a stimulus is, for example, frequently encoded by the number of receptors excited. This encoding, too, can be quantified, much as in the case of the intensity of a point stimulus. Further relevant characteristics are, for example, the site of a stimulus on the peripheral sensory area and the wavelengths of light (color) and of sound (pitch). Quantification of information in various regions of the nervous system is important, for example, when comparing objective neurophysiological findings with results of psychophysical measurements, for example, on the discrimination of stimuli.

Noise and redundancy in the transmission of information in the nervous system. The number of distinguishable levels of stimulus intensity calculated theoretically in the preceding section and the corresponding information capacity is not attained in reality. This statement is based on the experimental finding that for the same stimulus intensity the discharge frequency of a receptor varies in successive measurements. Figure 7-21A shows the discharge of a pressure receptor in the foot of a cat at various levels of stimulus intensity. As the pressure increases, the mean discharge frequency increases. It will also be noticed that, although the stimuli are constant with respect to time, the discharge rates are irregular. The discharge frequency, which is here the carrier of information about "stimulus intensity", fluctuates for no apparent reason. This fluctuation of the information carrier is called noise by the communications engineer, and it always means a reduction in the capacity of a communications channel, disturbing transmission. The noise associated with encoding in the receptor is also apparent in Fig. 7-21B. Each point denotes the result of a single measurement as in Fig. 7-21A. The number of impulses per second (ordinate) is plotted against the stimulus intensity (abscissa). At a stimulus intensity of, for example, 100 g the number of impulses determined in different measurements varies between about 32 and 41 per second.

The fluctuations in discharge frequency mean that the number of stimulus states that can be recognized by the receptor is smaller than one would expect theoretically on the basis of the maximum impulse rate, F_{max}. In the example given in Fig. 7-21B, the number of distin-

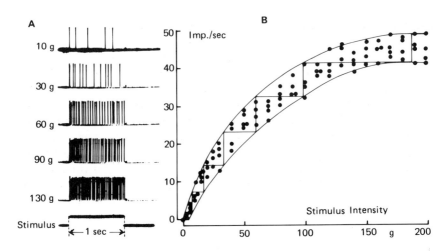

Fig. 7-21. Noise accompanying encoding in the receptor. *A* shows the original recordings of the discharge of a pressure receptor in a cat's paw for stimuli of 1 sec duration. The intensity of the stimulus increases from top to bottom. In *B* the measurements of the mean discharge frequency determined from many individual experiments of the type illustrated in *A* are plotted as a function of the stimulus intensity. The points of the individual measurements exhibit a range of scatter (bounded by the two curves). Because of these statistical fluctuations (noise) the number of intensity levels that can be discerned (as per the stepped curve shown) is less than theoretically possible according to Fig. 7-20.

guishable states, given stimulus durations of 1 sec, should be about 50, in accordance with what has been said before (see Fig. 7-1); however, the stepped curve shown in Fig. 7-21*B* has only eight steps (the first step is at 0 impulses per second). The corresponding values expressed in terms of information units are $\log_2 50 = 5.7$ bits/stimulus (theoretical) and $\log_2 8 = 3$ bits/stimulus (actual receptor). Thus 5.7 minus 3 bits = 2.7 bits of information are lost per stimulus as a result of noise. The resolution of the receptor when encoding the stimulus intensity is thus much less sharp than in the ideal case described in the preceding section.

Corresponding losses of information as a result of noise also occur in the case of each synaptic transmission of impulse trains. There are at least three synapses between the receptor and the sensory cortex. In order to be certain that information still reaches the brain despite repeated disturbances, the same information is encoded *simultaneously* in several fibers. The density of the receptors in the periphery is, in general, so high that even single-point stimuli excite several fibers in the same way. Since it is always the case that several fibers carrying the same information converge on the same neuron, a certain reserve of information is available that to a large extent compensates for the loss through noise. This parallel encoding of the information, which at first seems quite superfluous, is called *redundancy*. An excess of information plays a role in practically every transmission of information (in biology and technology). Redundancy protects the transmission of information from disturbance and loss. This is illustrated by Fig. 7-22. Here, you can recognize the information content of the sentence even though about 36 percent of the letters are missing. That is to say, written language contains more symbols than are strictly necessary for the sake of recognition. Language is thus redundant, and as a result it is protected against information losses. Redundancy is also measurable in bits.

In t..s c.apt.. t.e n..ve .s
co.par.d w.t. a tel.pho.. c.b l.

Fig. 7-22. Redundancy of written language. Despite the missing letters it is possible to recognize the information content of the text. Language does not utilize the maximum possible information content of the symbols (letters), and it is therefore redundant.

To stay with the example of language, linguistic studies with systematically mutilated texts have shown that written German utilizes on the average only 1.5 bits per letter. The redundancy is therefore 4.7 bits minus 1.5 bits = 3.2 bits per letter. In many books and scientific articles the redundancy is frequently even greater than this, often to the despair of the reader. An American journalist gave some of his younger colleagues a good tip on how to avoid such unnecessary verbosity: "Gentlemen," he said, "write every article as if you were going to wire it at your own expense to Australia!" But this is only one side of redundancy. Its advantages come to the fore when the channel is not clear, for example, a poor telephone connection, atmospherics on the radio, or illegible handwriting. In this case the redundancy of language ensures that even if only a fraction of the symbols is identifiable the text can be deciphered. It is a general tenet of information theory that as the encoding of a message becomes more redundant, it is less likely that the message will be lost during transmission. A very direct and effective means of providing redundancy is to transmit the message simultaneously along two or more channels. This is what happens in the nervous system as was shown above for the afferent fibers coming from the receptors.

Redundancy as a result of convergence and divergence; lateral inhibition. The principle of information transmission along several parallel fibers (in communications engineering this is referred to as multichannel transmission) is also retained after the synaptic relaying of the afferent fibers. The information about a stimulus is carried in several axons within an ascending bundle. These parallel pathways are, in addition, interconnected as we know from Chapter 4: each nerve fiber branches before synaptic relaying and forms synapses with several neurons (principle of divergence), and each neuron is linked with several presynaptic fibers (convergence). Analysis of these properties in terms of communications engineering shows that they render the transmission of information in the CNS even more redundant, but as a result the system is less prone to disturbance.

The protection against disturbance which is afforded by parallel transmission and interconnection of the parallel transmission paths (divergence and convergence) should really result in an excess of impulses as the information is transmitted up through the CNS. As indicated in Fig. 7-23A, the excitation should spread like an avalanche. However, this situation only occurs under pathological conditions, for example, when the CNS has been poisoned by strychnine. Then, even the slightest peripheral stimulus triggers a massive chain reaction of neuronal activity (strychnine convulsions). Strychnine has this effect because it eliminates *inhibition*. Inhibition is obviously a stabilizing factor in the nervous system. It operates in a manner similar to the

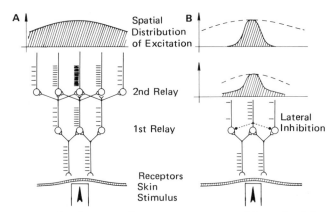

Fig. 7-23. Redundancy in the nervous sytem and lateral inhibition. Multichannel transmission, convergence, and divergence are characteristics that render information transmission in the nervous system redundant and thus less prone to disruption. However, the result is also that excitation spreads to such an extent in the CNS (A) that the image of the periphery is not sharply reproduced in the CNS. This lack of sharpness is compensated for neuronally (B) by the function of lateral inhibition at all the synaptic relays. Lateral inhibition is a predominant inhibitory effect exerted by the most strongly excited neuron on its surroundings (as denoted by the dotted connecting lines in B).

circuits known in communications and control engineering as *negative feedback*. Many neuronal inhibitory effects can be understood and described as negative feedback functions.

In particular, the spreading of the excitation shown in Fig. 7-23A is compensated for by a spatial arrangement of inhibitory connections known as *lateral inhibition*. This is illustrated in Fig. 7-23B. After the first synaptic relay the excitation exerts an inhibitory effect on the surrounding area via the interneurons (indicated by the dotted connecting lines in Fig. 7-23B). The most strongly excited neuron in the center (Fig. 7-23B) exerts a particularly strong inhibitory effect on its less excited surroundings. Conversely, the less strongly excited surroundings also have an inhibitory effect on the strongly excited center. However, for the sake of clarity this lesser effect has been omitted from Fig. 7-23B. Similar lateral inhibition also occurs in the subsequent synaptic relays. As a result, the spatial spreading of excitation in the CNS is limited as the shaded sections in Fig. 7-23B show in contrast to A. The excitation of central neurons by a stimulus can be regarded as image forming. In Fig. 7-23A the reproduction of the stimulus in the CNS is unresolved, blurred. By means of lateral inhibition (Fig. 7-23B) this lack of spatial resolution is compensated for, and this process is referred to as the *enhancement of spatial contrast*. This ability of the CNS is of great importance for all sensory systems.

Answer the following questions to check your knowledge.

Q 7.15 When the information "stimulus intensity" is encoded in the receptor, the information content can be calculated as
  a. the number of distinguishable states in the discharge frequency of the receptor.
  b. the number of action potentials generated per unit time.
  c. the logarithm to base 2 of the states of stimulus intensity which are distinguishable in the discharge of the receptor.
  d. Given random fluctuations in the discharge rate (noise), it is not possible to determine the information content.

Q 7.16 Which of the following statements about redundancy are correct? (More than one answer is correct.)
  a. Redundancy, generally speaking, involves an increase in effort above the necessary minimum level to transmit information.
  b. Redundancy is an increase in the information capacity of a nerve fiber, while at the same time the refractory period is shortened.
  c. Redundancy is achieved in the nervous system by transmitting the same information along several parallel pathways.
  d. With the redundancy of a neural message its proneness to disturbances also generally increases.

Q 7.17 Lateral inhibition in the CNS causes (more than one answer is correct)
    a.   compensation of the spread of excitation resulting from divergence.
    b.   complete suppression of all impulses generated by stimulation.
    c.   enhancement of spatial contrast and shaping of contours.
    d.   antagonistic inhibition of motoneurons.

8

THE AUTONOMIC
NERVOUS SYSTEM

The organism communicates with its environment by means of its somatic nervous system: the sensory system receives and processes information from the environment, and the motor system provides the means for getting about in the environment. The processes in the somatic nervous system are subject, for the most part, to conscious and voluntary control.

The autonomic nervous system behaves in a quite different way. It innervates the smooth musculature of all organs and systems of organs, the heart, and the glands. It regulates breathing, circulation, digestion, metabolism, secretions, body temperature, and reproduction and coordinates all these vital functions. As its name implies, the autonomic nervous system—sometimes also called the *vegetative* or the *involuntary* nervous system—is ordinarily not subject to direct voluntary control.

In functional terms, the actions of the autonomic and the somatic nervous systems are frequently inseparable. The functions of respiration and reproduction, for example, involve the participation of both the somatic and the autonomic nervous system.

8.1 Functional Anatomy of the Peripheral Autonomic Nervous System and of its Spinal Reflex Centers

The autonomic nervous system consists of two functionally different parts: the *sympathetic* and the *parasympathetic* systems. The terminal neurons of both systems, which correspond to the motoneurons in the somatic nervous system, are located outside the CNS. The

233

accumulations of the cell bodies of such neurons are called autonomic ganglia. The neuron that has its cell body in the CNS and terminates with its axon in such a ganglion is called a *preganglionic* neuron. The neuron that has its cell body in the ganglion and terminates with its axon on effectors is called a *postganglionic* neuron (see Fig. 8-1B, C).

In this section both portions of the autonomic nervous system are distinguished from each other with the aid of the following three important criteria: the origins of the preganglionic neurons in the CNS, the topographical position of the ganglia, and the chemical transmitter substances acting on the effectors (reacting organs).

The peripheral sympathetic system. The cell bodies of all preganglionic sympathetic neurons are located in the *thoracic* and the *upper lumbar spinal cord* (black shading in Fig. 8-1A). The axons of these neurons (solid lines in Fig. 8-2) leave the spinal cord in the ventral roots and run to the autonomic ganglia situated *outside the CNS*. The axons of the preganglionic neurons are relayed in the sympathetic ganglia to the cell bodies of the postganglionic neurons. The sympathetic ganglia are located in the region of the thoracic, the lumbar, and the sacral spinal cord (*Th, L, S* in Fig. 8-3A) and are organized segmentally to the left and the right of the spinal column.

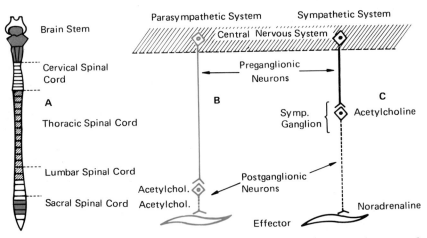

Fig. 8-1. Arrangement and transmitter substances of preganglionic and postganglionic neurons. *A*: Origins of the preganglionic neurons of the parasympathetic system (red) and of the sympathetic system (black shading) in the CNS. *B, C*: Diagrammatic view of the preganglionic and the postganglionic parasympathetic (*B*) and sympathetic (*C*) neurons. The axons of the preganglionic neurons are denoted by the solid lines and those of the postganglionic neurons by the dotted lines. The synaptic transmitter substances acting in the ganglia and on the effectors are shown.

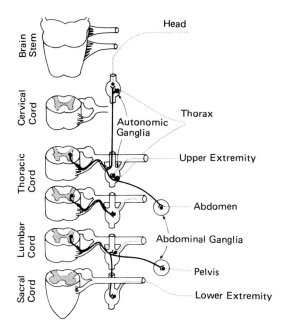

Fig. 8-2. Structure and innervation areas of the sympathetic system. The preganglionic axons are denoted by the solid lines, the postganglionic axons by the dotted lines. The autonomic ganglia are drawn too large in relation to the spinal cord segments.

In the region of the cervical cord (*C* in Fig. 8-3*A*) there are only two paired ganglia. The ganglia, which are arranged segmentally in pairs to the left and the right of the vertebral column, are connected from top to bottom by nerve trunks. These chains of ganglia are called the right and the left *sympathetic trunks* (Fig. 8-3*A*). In addition to these paired ganglia, there are unpaired ganglia in the abdominal and the pelvic regions in which the axons of the preganglionic neurons from both halves of the spinal cord terminate (Fig. 8-2). The preganglionic axons of these ganglia run through the sympathetic trunk ganglia without being relayed.

In the paired and the unpaired *ganglia* a preganglionic axon diverges on to many postganglionic cells, and many preganglionic neurons converge on a postganglionic cell. This is illustrated in Fig. 8-3*B*, in which the interconnections of four preganglionic axons and four postganglionic neurons in two ganglia are shown. The preganglionic axon *1* in the upper ganglion diverges onto the postganglionic cells *a*, *b*, and *c*. In the lower ganglion the three preganglionic axons *2*, *3*, and *4* converge on the postganglionic neuron *d*. As a result of this circuitry of the preganglionic and the postganglionic neurons, the activity of a

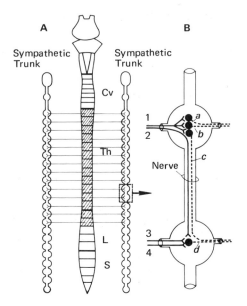

Fig. 8-3. Sympathetic trunk. *A:* Position of the left and the right sympathetic trunks in relation to spinal cord and brain stem. The ganglia are drawn too large in relation to the spinal cord segments. *Cv,* cervical cord; *Th,* thoracic cord; *L,* lumbar cord; *S,* sacral cord. *B:* Divergence (*1* onto *a, b,* and *c*) and convergence (*2, 3,* and *4* onto *d*) of preganglionic axons onto postganglionic neurons in the sympathetic trunk ganglia.

few preganglionic neurons is transmitted to many postganglionic neurons, and an individual postganglionic neuron receives the activity of many preganglionic neurons. This type of circuitry is an important safety factor guaranteeing ganglionic synaptic transmission.

Most preganglionic sympathetic fibers are myelinated. They are less than 4 μ in diameter. Thus they propagate the excitation at speeds below 20 m/sec. The postganglionic fibers are very thin and unmyelinated. Their propagation speed is less than 1 m/sec.

The axons of the postganglionic neurons (black dotted lines in Fig. 8-2) emerge from the ganglia and innervate the effectors of the sympathetic system. The postganglionic neurons, on which preganglionic neurons from the thoracic spinal cord converge, innervate the head, the thorax, the abdomen, and the upper extremities. The postganglionic neurons on which preganglionic neurons from the lumbar spinal cord converge, innervate the pelvis and the lower extremities (Fig. 8-2). The ganglia of the sympathetic system are usually relatively far removed from the reacting organs; therefore the postganglionic sympathetic axons are often very long (Fig. 8-1*C,* 8-2). The effectors of

The peripheral parasympathetic system. The cell bodies of the preganglionic neurons of the peripheral parasympathetic nervous system are located in the *sacral cord* and the *brain stem*. The preganglionic parasympathetic fibers are, for the most part, unmyelinated and, as indicated in Fig. 8-1*B*, are very long in contrast to the preganglionic sympathetic fibers because the parasympathetic ganglia are located in the vicinity of the effectors. The parasympathetic axons from the brain stem run in the *vagus nerve* to the organs in the thorax and the abdomen (solid red lines in Fig. 8-4) and in other cranial nerves to the

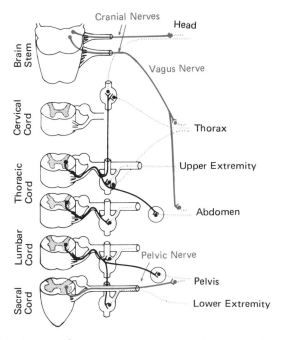

Fig. 8-4. Structure and innervation areas of the sympathetic and the parasympathetic systems. Similar diagram as in Fig. 8-2. Here, in addition, the pre- and the postganglionic neurons of the parasympathetic system are shown in red.

organs of the head. The fibers from the sacral cord run in the pelvic nerve to the organs in the pelvis (Fig. 8-4). The autonomic ganglia in which preganglionic and postganglionic parasympathetic neurons are interconnected are distributed in the walls of the effectors or in the vicinity of the effectors. The postganglionic parasympathetic fibers (red dotted lines in Fig. 8-4) are therefore very short in comparison with the corresponding sympathetic fibers (black dotted lines in Fig. 8-4). All the parasympathetically innervated organs, such as the bladder, the rectum (pelvic region), the gastrointestinal tract (abdomen), the heart, the lungs (thorax), and the lacrimal and the salivary glands (head region) are also innervated by sympathetic fibers. However, not all sympathetically innervated organs are innervated by the parasympathetic system. In particular, this is true of the entire vascular system (arteries, veins).

The synaptic transmitter substances in the peripheral autonomic nervous system. In Chapter 3 you learned that the transmission of impulses between two neurons as well as between a neuron and the effector is mostly chemically mediated. Likewise in the peripheral autonomic nervous system chemical synapses also exist between preganglionic and postganglionic neurons and between postganglionic neurons and effectors. At these synapses the excitation is transmitted by the release of chemical agents. The transmitters from the postganglionic neurons to most effectors are different in the sympathetic and the parasympathetic systems. This is therefore a further distinguishing characteristic of these two divisions of the autonomic nervous system. In the sympathetic and the parasympathetic ganglia the synaptic transmitter from the preganglionic axons to the postganglionic cells is *acetylcholine* (Fig. 8-1B,C). The transmission is cholinergic, as it is at the muscle end plate.

As in the ganglia, the parasympathetic transmitter to the effectors is also *acetylcholine* (Fig. 8-1B). For this reason, the parasympathetic system is also called the *cholinergic system*. The transmitter from the postganglionic axons of the sympathetic system to the effectors is, with one exception, *noradrenaline* (norepinephrine). Therefore, the sympathetic nervous system is also called, after its transmitter substance, the *adrenergic system*. The exception is in the case of the sweat gland fibers. They transmit their activity to the sweat glands by releasing acetylcholine. These fibers are therefore cholinergic.

The medulla of the suprarenal gland plays a special role in the body. It is a transformed sympathetic ganglion and consists of modified postganglionic neurons. When the preganglionic neurons that innervate the suprarenal medulla are excited, these postganglionic

...visceral afferents. So far, we have discussed the efferents of the autonomic nervous system. There are, however, also afferents that are sometimes assigned to the autonomic nervous system. These come from the visceral region and are therefore called visceral afferents (see also Fig. 1-8). Even though the visceral afferents that run in the vagus nerve and the pelvic nerve are called parasympathetic afferents, it is not possible technically to make a clear functional and morphological distinction between sympathetic and parasympathetic afferents.

The receptors of the visceral afferents are situated in the organs of the thorax, the abdomen, and the pelvis, and also in the walls of the blood vessels. These receptors measure the intraluminal pressure (for example, in the arterial system) or the degree of fullness of the hollow organs (for example, the bladder, the veins, the intestine) indirectly by the stretching of the walls of the hollow organs. They also record the acidity and the electrolytic concentration of the contents of the hollow organs (for example, of the blood or the stomach contents) and also pain stimuli in the visceral region. Like the somatic afferents, the visceral afferents enter the spinal cord in the dorsal roots. They have their cell bodies in the spinal ganglia. A large number of the visceral afferents from the abdomen and the thorax run in the vagus nerve. Their cell bodies are situated in an appropriate sensory ganglion below the base of the skull.

You should now be able to answer the following questions.

Q 8.1 The sympathetic and the parasympathetic autonomic peripheral nervous systems can be distinguished according to the
    a. origins of the preganglionic neurons.
    b. synaptic transmitters in the autonomic ganglia.
    c. position of the autonomic ganglia.
    d. synaptic transmitters acting on the effectors.
    e. organs that they innervate in the thorax and the abdomen.

Q 8.2 Which of the following statements apply to the peripheral parasympathetic nervous system?
    a. It controls the hormonal balance.
    b. It has long preganglionic neurons.
    c. It innervates only the organs in the head, the thorax, the abdomen, and the pelvis.
    d. It transmits excitation to the effectors with acetylcholine.

    e. It consists of preganglionic and postganglionic neurons that
       are connected in the sympathetic trunk.
    f. It innervates all organs that are also innervated by the sympa-
       thetic system.

Q 8.3 In which of the following are the cell bodies of the preganglionic
    neurons of the sympathetic nervous system situated?
    a. Effectors.
    b. Sympathetic trunk.
    c. Thoracic spinal cord.
    d. Sacral spinal cord.
    e. Lumbar spinal cord.
    f. Mesencephalon (midbrain).

Q 8.4 The visceral afferents
    a. have their cell bodies in the sympathetic trunk.
    b. enter the CNS with the somatic afferents.
    c. come from the intestinal and the vascular region.
    d. have their cell bodies in the spinal ganglia or in the sensory
       ganglion of the vagus nerve.
    e. make synapses outside the CNS.

8.2 The Reactions of the Smooth Muscle to Stretching, Acetylcholine, Noradrenaline, and Neural Stimulation

The autonomic nervous system innervates all the smooth muscles
of the body. In this section a description will be given of some of the
identifying features of smooth muscle based on the special characteristics of the cell membrane and the structure of the smooth muscle.
With the aid of these features it is possible to explain the way in which
many autonomically innervated organs function. We will first see that
when a smooth muscle cell is stretched, it depolarizes, and this depolarization triggers a contraction. A description will then be given of
the actions of noradrenaline and acetylcholine on a stretched intestinal muscle. Finally, the contractions of a smooth muscle and a skeletal
muscle after neural stimulation will be compared.

The development of force by smooth muscle cells on stretching.
The smooth muscles of an organ consist of single fusiform cells that
are about 50 to 200 μ long and 5 to 10 μ thick. The cells are interconnected in reticular fashion. Smooth muscle cells, like skeletal muscle
cells, contain myofibrils, although in far smaller quantities. These
myofibrils are not regularly arranged as in the skeletal muscle, so it is
not possible to detect any striation in the smooth muscles. The con-

tl
in
the
very
stret
when
curve ⌐ ... ...usue in contrast to that of skeletal muscle (see Fig. 3-3) is thus much less steep.

Figure 8-5 shows a test arrangement for measuring the force developed by an intestinal muscle and also the membrane potential of a single cell of this preparation. The intestinal muscle is immersed in a bath solution. The muscle can be stretched passively (right in figure). The force the preparation develops during stretching is measured isometrically with a force meter (left in figure). The membrane potential of a single smooth muscle cell is measured intracellularly with a microelectrode.

Figure 8-6,I shows a preparation of intestinal muscle in a state of stretch such as might be encountered in a living, moderately filled organ. In this stretched state, the smooth musculature of the intestine is *spontaneously active*; that is, the cell membranes of the smooth muscle cells depolarize without the action of external stimuli. If these depolarizations reach the threshold, they generate propagated action potentials. The membrane potential of a single cell of the preparation in Fig. 8-6A,I is approximately −50 mV (Fig. 8-6B,I). From this potential an action potential is generated approximately every 1.2 sec.

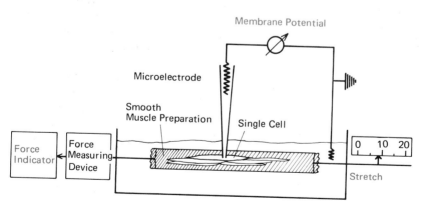

Fig. 8-5. Diagrammatic view of a test arrangement for recording the membrane potential and the active development of force of smooth muscle cells when passively stretched. It is in principle the same setup as that illustrated in Fig. 3-3. To the right, the muscle preparation is pretensioned; to the left, the force is measured isometrically.

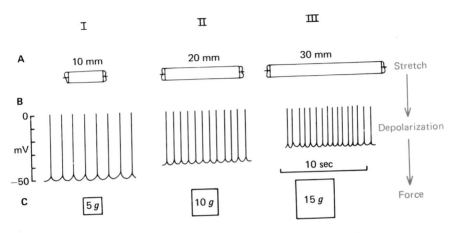

Fig. 8-6. Force developed by a preparation of intestinal muscle upon stretching. *A*: Stretching of the preparation by 10 and 20 mm. At zero the preparation has the same degree of tension that it would have *in situ* in the intestine. *B*: Membrane potential of a single cell of the muscle preparation. *C*: Force developed by the preparation.

These spontaneous action potentials are generated in many cells of the preparation. At the same time, the entire specimen of intestinal muscle develops a force of 5 g (Fig. 8-6*C,I*). Stretching of the preparation by 10 mm (Fig. 8-6*A,II*) lowers the membrane potential of the cell of the preparation (Fig. 8-6*B,II*). The frequency of the action potentials propagating along the length of the cell increases. At the same time the preparation develops a force of 10 g. Stretching the preparation another 10 mm results in a further decrease in membrane potential of the smooth muscle cell and an increase in the frequency of the action potentials and the force developed by the preparation (Fig. 8-6,*III A–C*).

If the generation of action potentials is prevented, no force is developed by the preparation, although the membrane potential drops on stretching. We can deduce from this that the stretching of a smooth muscle depolarizes its fiber membrane. This depolarization triggers propagated action potentials, which in turn give rise to the generation of force by the preparation. As in the case of skeletal muscle, contraction of smooth muscle cells is triggered by action potentials propagating across the fibers. The relationships between membrane potential (MP), frequency of the action potentials (AP/10 sec), and development of force (force) are shown quantitatively in Fig. 8-7 for the preparation illustrated in Fig. 8-6. *A* shows the relationship between discharge frequency (abscissa) and membrane potential (ordinate). *B* shows the relationship between the development of force

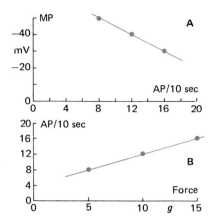

Fig. 8-7. Relationships between membrane potential and discharge frequency (A) and between discharge frequency and development of force (B) of a preparation of intestinal muscle. The membrane potential (MP) in millivolts, the discharge frequency in action potentials/10 sec (AP/10 sec), and the force in g were taken from Fig. 8-6A–C.

by the preparation (abscissa) and the discharge frequency of a cell (ordinate). Clearly the discharge frequency of the cell is inversely proportional to its membrane potential and directly proportional to the force developed by the entire preparation. From this test we can conclude that the extent to which force is developed by a smooth muscle is determined by the degree of depolarization of the fiber membranes of its individual cells.

The action potentials of a smooth muscle cell are also propagated electrotonically across the cell boundaries to neighboring cells. It is assumed that this occurs by means of contact points between the cells that offer low resistance to propagation. The result of this propagation of the action potentials is that a large number of muscle cells can be made to contract by the depolarization of a single muscle cell. For example, if the excitation threshold in only one in a population of smooth muscle cells is particularly low, then this cell can initiate contraction in the surrounding cells. This muscle cell is called the *pacemaker* for the surrounding cells. In principle every cell in a smooth muscle is capable of acting as a pacemaker for its surroundings.

The increasing excitability arising from stretching of the membranes of the smooth muscle cells is of great importance for the hollow organs of the body, such as the intestine, the blood vessels, and the bladder. Any increase in the filling of a hollow organ generates increased activity in its wall muscles. Thus, for example, if nervous control of the bladder is lost as a result of destruction of the sacral spinal cord, the bladder will nevertheless empty itself spontaneously once it has filled to a certain point. The intrinsic excitability of the smooth muscles and its modification by mechanical stretching enable the hollow organs to perform their functions to a limited extent without nervous control. In this connection we talk of the *autonomy* of the vegetatively (autonomically) innervated organs.

Besides these spontaneously active smooth muscles there are certain classes of smooth muscles whose cells are in general neither spontaneously active nor depolarized by mechanical stretching. These are, for example, the smooth muscles associated with hairs and those that adjust the lens of the eye. These muscles can only be activated by the autonomic nerves that serve them.

The direct effects of acetylcholine and noradrenaline on smooth muscle cells.   Smooth muscles can be influenced directly by a large number of drugs. It is for this reason that smooth muscles are frequently used as biological test objects in many pharmacological assays. In the following, the effects of acetylcholine and adrenaline on a resting (pretensioned) preparation of intestinal smooth muscle will be described.

The test arrangement is the same as in Fig. 8-5. A preparation of intestinal muscle is immersed under tension in a bath solution. The membrane potential of a smooth muscle cell and the force developed by this preparation are measured.

The upper trace in Fig. 8-8A shows the membrane potential (MP) of a single pretensioned smooth muscle cell from the intestine. The membrane potential in this cell is about -50 mV. The beginning of the intracellular recording shows that as a result of the pretensioning the cell depolarizes to the threshold and thus continuously triggers action potentials. The lower trace in Figure 8-8A shows the force developed by the entire preparation. At the start of the measurement with the preparation at rest, the force developed amounts to about 1 g. When a very small quantity of acetylcholine is added to the bath solution (black bar in Fig. 8-8A), the membrane of the muscle cell depolarizes, and the frequency of the action potentials along the muscle fiber increases. At the same time the force developed by the preparation increases to 3 g. When the acetylcholine solution is replaced by a normal bath solution (last third of the trace in Fig. 8-8A) the MP returns to its initial value. The tension of the preparation decreases again as a result of the reduced frequency of the propagated action potentials.

As shown by this experiment, acetylcholine triggers reactions in

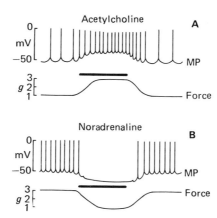

Fig. 8-8. Reaction of smooth muscle cells to acetylcholine (*A*) and noradrenaline (*B*). Test setup as in Fig. 8-5. The preparation of intestinal muscle is pretensioned. The upper curves in *A* and *B* depict the membrane potential (MP) of a muscle cell of the preparation, and the lower curves depict the force developed by the entire preparation. During the time denoted by the thick black line, the preparation was bathed in a solution of acetylcholine or noradrenaline.

the smooth muscles of the intestine comparable to those induced by mechanical stretching. It is assumed that both stretching of the cell membranes and the action of acetylcholine increase the membrane conductance for the same ions, particularly Na^+ ions, depolarizing these membranes.

The effect of a dilute solution of noradrenaline on a preparation of intestinal muscle is illustrated in Fig. 8-8*B*. As a result of the pretensioning the preparation develops a force of 3 g. Noradrenaline (thick black line in *B*) increases the potential of the muscle cell membranes. The cell from which the recording is made in Fig. 8-8*B* hyperpolarizes, and no more propagated action potentials are generated. As a result, the force developed by the preparation declines, and the preparation becomes flaccid. During stretching, noradrenaline impedes the depolarization of the intestinal muscle cell membranes and thus the contractions of the muscle cells.

Noradrenaline has an inhibitory effect on the smooth muscles of the intestines and the lungs. Other smooth muscles, for example, the vascular muscles, are excited by noradrenaline. Acetylcholine has an excitatory effect on the smooth muscles of the intestine and the lung.

Comparison of contractions of a smooth and a striated muscle after neural stimulation. So far we have considered the behavior of the smooth muscles independent of their autonomic innervation. In the following, the contraction of a smooth muscle after stimulation of an autonomic nerve will be compared with the contraction of a skeletal muscle. It is known from electron-microscope and physiological tests that neuromuscular transmission in smooth muscle is qualitatively the same as that in skeletal muscle. However, there are certain quantitative differences. The autonomic nerve fibers do not always terminate with morphologically distinct neuromuscular synapses on the smooth muscle cells; instead, the axons pass adjacent to the smooth muscle cells at various distances. The transmitter substance is released from the axons and diffuses to the smooth muscle cells. It is assumed that the transmitter substance of an autonomic terminal axon acts on many smooth muscle cells in its vicinity. The postsynaptic excitatory potentials that can be measured in muscle cells after neural stimulation last about 10 to 20 times longer than the end-plate potentials in skeletal muscle fibers. In some muscle cells (for example, those of the intestine) it is also possible to measure inhibitory postsynaptic potentials running in a hyperpolarizing direction after stimulation of the sympathetic nerves.

Figure 8-9 shows nerve-muscle preparations of a skeletal muscle (left) and a smooth muscle (right). The smooth muscle is the sympathetically innervated muscle of the nictitating membrane of the eye of a cat. The nerve action potential (C,F), the muscle action potential (B,E), and the muscle contraction (A,D) of each preparation were measured after stimulation of the nerves with electrodes, R. When the

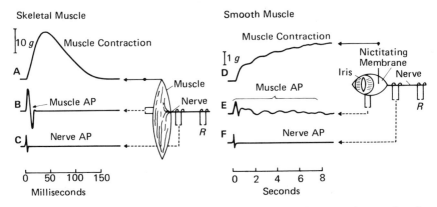

Fig. 8-9. Contraction of a skeletal muscle and of a smooth muscle after neural stimulation. The smooth muscle is the sympathetically innervated muscle of the nictitating membrane of the eye of a cat. The nerve action potential (C,F), the muscle action potential (B,E), and the contraction of the muscle (A,D) are recorded after stimulation of the nerve via electrodes, R. Note the different time scales. (Modified from Ruch and Patton, Physiology and Biophysics, Philadelphia and London, Saunders Company, 1965.)

nerve of the skeletal muscle is stimulated, a short-lasting nerve action potential (C) is recorded extracellularly in the same nerve. It is composed of the action potentials of individual fibers. Shortly after the start of the nerve action potential a muscle action potential (mass action potential) lasting about 10 to 15 msec is recorded in the muscle (B). After a delay of a few milliseconds, this is followed by a contraction of the skeletal muscle (A). The contraction of the skeletal muscle increases within about 30 msec to its maximum value and lasts for about 150 msec. If the nerve to the smooth muscle of the nictitating membrane is stimulated (Fig. 8-9, right), this also leads to a short-lasting nerve action potential (F). This potential is followed by a long-lasting muscle action potential (E) that is composed of several components (note the different time scales for the right and the left diagrams). Contraction of the smooth muscle, in contrast to that of the skeletal muscle, begins with a noticeable delay after the start of the nerve and the muscle action potentials (D). The contraction increases slowly and attains its maximum after about 8 sec.

It is typical of smooth muscles that their electrical (E) and mechanical activity (D) last longer than the excitatory nerve action potential (F). This behavior can be attributed in part to the structure of the smooth muscles. Also, however, the chemical transmitter substance that is released by the nerve endings acts longer on the smooth muscle cells because it is not broken down so quickly by enzymes as it is in the motor end plate of the skeletal muscle.

In order to attain a lasting contraction of the skeletal muscle (tetanus) the nerve of the muscle must be excited with approximately 100 stimuli per second (see Sec. 5.2). In the case of the long-lasting, slowly increasing and decreasing contraction of the smooth muscle, considerably lower stimulus frequencies of about 2 to 3 impulses/sec are required to generate a uniform contraction of the muscle. Thus, relatively low frequencies of 2 to 3 action potentials per second in the efferent autonomic fibers are sufficient to achieve a certain uniform state of contraction (tonus) in the smooth muscle.

Q 8.5 Stretching of a preparation of smooth muscle from the intestine
  a. results in depolarization of the membrane of the smooth muscle cells.
  b. brings about a reduction in the discharge frequency of the smooth muscle cells.
  c. leads to relaxation of the muscle preparation.
  d. causes the muscle preparation to develop force.
  e. increases the membrane potential.

Q 8.6 The graded development of force by a smooth muscle (intestine)

    a. is controlled by the depolarization of the fiber membranes of the muscle cells.
    b. can be triggered by bathing the preparation in variously diluted solutions of adrenaline.
    c. is impossible because the contraction of the smooth muscle is an all-or-nothing event.
    d. can be triggered by acetylcholine solution.   ·
    e. can be generated by mechanical stretching of the muscle.

Q 8.7 What is the relationship between development of force, K, membrane potential, M, and action potential frequency, F, in a smooth muscle?
    a. K is directly proportional to M.
    b. K is directly proportional to F.
    c. F is inversely proportional to M.
    d. F is proportional to M.

Q 8.8 The contraction of a smooth muscle after neural stimulation
    a. is an event lasting _____ (tens of msec/100 msec/seconds).
    b. lasts about _____ (2/5/100) times longer than the contraction of a skeletal muscle.
    c. increases _____ (more quickly than/at the same rate as/more slowly than) that of a skeletal muscle.
    d. starts _____ (later than/at the same time as/earlier than) that of a skeletal muscle.
    e. is caused by _____ (the same/different) basic mechanisms.

8.3 The Antagonistic Effects of Sympathetic and Parasympathetic Activity on the Autonomic Effectors

Most autonomically innervated organs are independently active; that is, they function even in the denervated state. Since the organs in question are almost exclusively hollow organs, such as the gastrointestinal tract, the bladder, and the blood vessels, their function is regulated by the degree of filling or the internal pressure. Increased internal pressure stretches the smooth muscles in the walls of the organ and depolarizes the membrane of the smooth muscle cells. This in turn leads to force being generated by the smooth musculature and thus to displacement of the contents of the hollow organ. This autonomous function of the organs can be traced back to the characteristics of the smooth musculature (see Sec. 8.2).

Most of these organs are innervated by sympathetic and parasympathetic fibers and visceral afferent fibers. The activity in the efferent autonomic fibers is superimposed on the autonomous activity of the organs. The sympathetic and the parasympathetic activities are mostly antagonistic in their effect on the organs. In the following, we will describe this antagonistic action on two examples—an intestinal muscle and a frog's heart. These specimens have been chosen to demonstrate nervous control of the digestive, the excretory, and the cardiovascular systems.

Autonomic influences on the heart. An isolated frog's heart continues to beat *spontaneously* without any connection whatsoever with the body. Like almost all other autonomically innervated organs the heart is *independently active.* The heart rate is controlled by a group of modified muscle cells situated at the entrance to the heart. These cells depolarize spontaneously and generate propagated action potentials that are transmitted by other specialized muscle cells to the muscles of the chambers of the heart, which pump the blood into the arterial system. In this way the contractions of separate areas of the heart are coordinated with one another. These spontaneously depolarizing cells at the entrance are called *pacemaker cells.* The autonomic nervous system acts on both the pacemaker cells and the other cardiac muscle cells.

Figure 8-10 (left) shows an isolated frog's heart. The heart rate and the contractile force of the heart are recorded mechanically at the apex of the heart by a pointer, P. The heart rate is given by the *frequency* of the pointer deflections, and the force of contraction is given by the

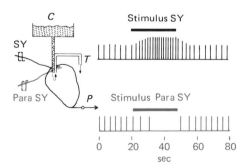

Fig. 8-10. Nervous control of the heart. To the left is a diagram of an isolated frog's heart whose sympathetic (SY) and parasympathetic (*Para SY*) nerves are attached to electrodes. The contractions of the heart are indicated by a pointer, P and recorded before, during, and after stimulation of the sympathetic nerve (upper record) and the parasympathetic nerve (lower record). Blood substitute solution runs into the heart from the container, C.

magnitude of the deflection (recording traces on right). The two autonomic nerves that innervate the heart, the sympathetic cardiac nerve and the parasympathetic cardiac nerve, are connected to stimulating electrodes. Blood substitute solution runs from the container, *C*, into the heart and is pumped out again through the tube, *T*.

At the start of the recording in Fig. 8-10 the heart beats spontaneously at a rate of about 18 beats per minute. When the *sympathetic nerve* is stimulated electrically (upper record) the time between the pointer deflections becomes shorter, and the magnitude of the deflection increases. This means that the *heart rate* and also the *contractile force* of the heart both *increase*. Once stimulation of the sympathetic nerve stops, the heart resumes its spontaneous rhythm. Excitation of the *parasympathetic nerve* (lower record) results in quite different changes in the autonomic activity of the heart. The time between the contractions of the heart increases until the heart comes to a standstill; in other words, the parasympathetic nerve *lowers* the *heart rate*. The magnitude of the deflections remains constant during electrical stimulation of the parasympathetic nerve. We can conclude from this that the parasympathetic activity does not influence directly the contractile force of the heart. The innervation regions of the parasympathetic and the sympathetic nerves in the heart correspond to the effects these nerves have on contractile force and heart rate. The sympathetic nerve innervates both the region in the atrial wall, which determines the heart rate (pacemaker cells), and also the muscles of the ventricles of the heart. The parasympathetic nerve innervates only the pacemaker cells and the atria of the heart.

The amount of blood pumped by the heart per unit time (*cardiac output*) depends on the heart rate and on the contractile force of the heart. Sympathetic activity increases the cardiac output; parasympathetic activity reduces it. Both portions of the nervous system thus have a mutually antagonistic effect on the spontaneously active heart. Of course, regulation of the cardiac output by the autonomic nervous system never occurs in the organism in the strict manner illustrated in Fig. 8-10 because the sympathetic and the parasympathetic systems influence the heart simultaneously. The heart is subjected continuously to inhibitory parasympthetic and excitatory sympathetic influences. Each change in activity in one or the other of the two autonomic systems results in changes in the heart rate and/or the contractile force. Thus the cardiac output (amount of blood pumped by the heart per unit time) increases when there is a rise in sympathetic activity and/or a drop in parasympathetic activity. The cardiac output declines when there is a drop in sympathetic activity and/or a rise in parasympathetic activity. Since the CNS has these means at its disposal to regulate the cardiac output through the autonomic nervous system, the body can adapt its cardiovascular system to the environmental requirements.

The chemical transmission of activity from the autonomic cardiac nerves to the heart. A frog's heart is a very suitable biological specimen for testing autonomic synaptic transmitter substances because its cells are very sensitive to these substances. Very small quantities are sufficient to evoke reactions in the test specimen. Figure 8-11 (left) shows diagrammatically the test arrangement that some time ago led to the discovery of chemical synaptic transmission from the autonomic fibers to the effectors in the frog's heart. The upper part of the test arrangement is the same as in Fig. 8-10. In addition, in Fig. 8-11 the blood substitute solution is pumped from heart I through the tube, T, to heart II.

The two upper records in Fig. 8-11 are the same as those in Fig. 8-10. Stimulation of the sympathetic cardiac nerve increases the rate of the heart beat and the contractile force of the heart. Stimulation of the parasympathetic cardiac nerve lowers the heart rate and provokes temporary cardiac arrest. The second heart, which is connected with heart I by the tube, T, beats spontaneously at a slightly faster rate than heart I. When the autonomic nerves of heart I are stimulated, the rate of the heart beat and the contractile force of heart II change in the same direction as in heart I. These changes in heart II occur with a clear delay after the changes have taken place in heart I. In addition, the changes are not so pronounced as in heart I.

It can be concluded from the results of this particular experiment

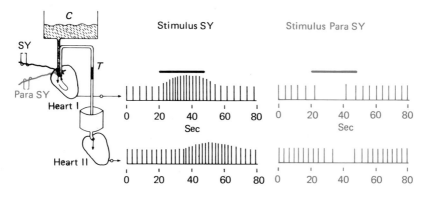

Fig. 8-11. Release of synaptic transmitter substances after stimulation of the autonomic cardiac nerves. The blood substitute solution is pumped from heart I to heart II. Otherwise the arrangement is as in Fig. 8-10.

that the changes in the rate and the contractile force of heart *II* are generated by substances released into the nutrient medium by heart *I* and passing through the tube, *T*, when the autonomic nerves of heart *I* are stimulated. This test proves beyond all doubt that the transmission from the terminals of the autonomic fibers to the heart is chemical. The effects of the chemical substances show, furthermore, that the sympathetic and the parasympathetic systems release different transmitters. The substances released alter the rate of the heart beat and the contractile force of the heart *II* just as if this heart had been directly influenced by autonomic nerves. It must be concluded that the substances released are the sympathetic and the parasympathetic transmitter substances.

Autonomic control of the intestinal musculature. Pronounced antagonistic effects of the sympathetic and the parasympathetic systems can also be observed in the entire digestive system. The following will show how the force developed by a specimen of intestinal muscle changes after stimulation of the sympathetic and the parasympathetic nerves that innervate the preparation. Simultaneously, the membrane potential in a smooth muscle cell of the specimen is measured. The experimental arrangement is the same as in Fig. 8-5. Figure 8-12A shows the effects of parasympathetic and sympathetic activity on the

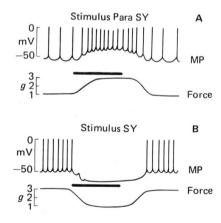

Fig. 8-12. Effects of the parasympathetic nerve (*A*) and the sympathetic nerve (*B*) on the smooth muscle cells of the intestine. The test arrangement is the same as in Fig. 8-5. The parasympathetic and the sympathetic nerves of the intestinal muscle preparation were left intact. The upper records in *A* and *B* show the membrane potential of a muscle cell of the preparation; the lower records show the force which the entire preparation develops. During the period marked by the heavy black line, the parasympathetic (*A*) and the sympathetic (*B*) nerves of the preparation were stimulated.

musculature of the intestines. When the parasympathetic nerve is stimulated, the membrane of the smooth muscle cell is depolarized (upper record in A). The frequency of the action potentials propagating along the fiber increases. As a result, the smooth muscle cells contract. The force developed by the entire preparation increases (lower record in A). Stimulation of the sympathetic nerve produces the opposite effects (B). The membrane of the cell hyperpolarizes, no more action potentials are generated, and consequently the intestinal muscle relaxes. These antagonistic effects of the sympathetic and the parasympathetic nerves on the intestinal musculature correspond to the direct effects of noradrenaline and acetylcholine, the autonomic transmitter substances, on the intestinal muscles (see Fig. 8-8).

The *same* transmitters of the autonomic nervous system have inhibitory or excitatory effects on the membranes depending on the effector. It is probable that these transmitters can increase the conductances of the membranes in a relatively selective fashion for potassium or sodium ions. These changes in conductance lead to shifts in the membrane potential of the cells in the direction of the potassium or the sodium equilibrium potential, and this results in hyperpolarization or depolarization of the cells, respectively.

Q 8.9 In Sec. 8-1 you learned that after excitation of the sympathetic system, mainly adrenaline is released into the bloodstream by the cells of the suprarenal medulla. What effect does this adrenaline produce?
   a. It increases the movement of the intestine.
   b. It reduces the contractile force of the heart.
   c. It inhibits intestinal function.
   d. It increases the cardiac output.
   e. It blocks cholinergic transmission from the parasympathetic system to the intestinal muscles.

Q 8.10 Which of the following statements are correct?
   a. Acetylcholine reduces cardiac output.
   b. Adrenaline increases the movements of the intestine.
   c. Acetylcholine decreases the movements of the intestine.
   d. Adrenaline increases the cardiac output.

Q 8.11 In which way can the CNS increase the volume of blood pumped per minute by the heart? (Think of the heart rate and the contractile force of the heart.)
   a. Increasing the activity in the sympathetic cardiac nerves.
   b. Decreasing the activity in the sympathetic cardiac nerves.
   c. Increasing the activity in the parasympathetic cardiac
   d. nerves.
      Decreasing the activity in the parasympathetic cardiac nerves.

8.4   Central Nervous Regulation of the Autonomic Effectors

The activity of autonomically innervated organs can be inhibited or increased by the sympathetic or the parasympathetic systems. The central relay stations that transmit these effects are located in the spinal cord and the brain stem. The efferents of these relay stations are essentially the sympathetic and the parasympathetic nerves; the afferent inputs originate both peripherally (visceral and sometimes somatic) and centrally (from higher autonomic centers). This section shows how the activity of the autonomically innervated organs is centrally regulated.

First we will discuss the autonomic reflex arc and the segmental circuitry of autonomic efferents and visceral and somatic afferents. Then we shall consider the spinal nervous regulation of the excretory system using the micturition reflex as an example. Finally, we shall outline the central nervous regulation of the cardiovascular circulation.

The spinal autonomic reflex arc. The simplest connection between afferents and autonomic efferents is situated at the segmental level in the spinal cord. This neuronal circuit is called the *autonomic reflex arc*. Fig. 8-13 shows a cross section through the spinal cord with the autonomic reflex arc on the left and the simplest somatic reflex arc (monosynaptic) on the right. The efferent neuron of the autonomic reflex arc that transmits its activity to the autonomic effectors is the postganglionic neuron (*b* in Fig. 8-13). Its soma is located outside the

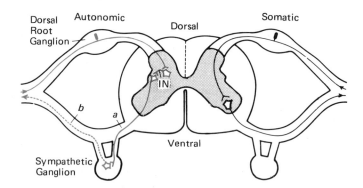

Fig. 8-13. Autonomic reflex arc (left) compared with a monosynaptic reflex arc (right). *IN* = interneuron; *a* = preganglionic neuron; *b* = postganglionic neuron.

spinal cord in an autonomic ganglion. The cell body of the efferent neuron of the somatic reflex arc is situated in the ventral horn of the spinal cord.

The afferent fibers of the autonomic reflex arc are both *visceral and somatic*, and they enter the spinal cord in the dorsal roots. At least two neurons are interposed between the afferent neuron and the postganglionic neuron: an interneuron (*IN* in Fig. 8-13) and the preganglionic neuron (*a* in Fig. 8-13). The monosynaptic reflex arc, on the other hand, contains no neuron between afferent fiber and motoneuron. The autonomic reflex arc thus has at least two synapses in the gray matter of the spinal cord and one synapse in the ganglion between preganglionic neuron and postganglionic neuron. The simplest somatic reflex arc has only one synapse between afferent and efferent neuron.

The segmental connection of autonomic efferents with visceral and somatic afferents. When pathological processes occur in the intestinal region (for example, cholecystitis or gastritis) it is noted that the muscles over the site of the disorder are taut. The skin that is innervated by afferents and efferents of the same spinal cord segment as the pathologically affected intestine (dermatome) is reddened. The "stomach ache," which is caused by the cramplike motions of the intestines, can be eased or even eliminated by changing the skin temperature of the dermatome (for example, by applying poultices) which is innervated by the same spinal cord segment as the affected intestine.

From these observations we must conclude that the visceral and the somatic afferents are connected with autonomic and somatic efferents at the segmental level of the spinal cord. Figure 8-14 is a cross section through the spinal cord with the reflex arcs responsible for (1) the reddening of the skin and the defensive tensioning of the skeletal muscle when pathological processes occur in the intestines and (2) the relief of the stomach ache by changing the temperataure of the skin. Not all the interneurons in the gray matter of the spinal cord have been included. A somatic afferent from the skin (*b* in Fig. 8-14) and a somatic efferent to the skeletal muscle (*e*) are shown in black. A visceral afferent from the intestine (*a*) and also one autonomic efferent to the intestine (*c*) and one to a cutaneous blood vessel (*d*) are shown in red. The *reddening* of the skin area is caused by dilation of the blood vessels in the skin. Thus, visceral afferents of the intestines (*a* in Fig. 8-14) must be connected with the autonomic (sympathetic) efferents to the cutaneous blood vessels (*d* in Fig. 8-14), the viscerocutaneous reflex. If, at the same time, the *abdominal muscles* over the

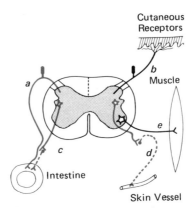

Fig. 8-14. Connection of autonomic and somatic efferents with somatic and visceral afferents at the segmental level. *a* visceral afferent from the intestine; *b* somatic afferent from thermoreceptors in the skin; *c* autonomic (sympathetic) efferent to the intestine; *d* autonomic (sympathetic) efferent to blood vessel in skin (vasoconstrictor); *e* somatic efferent to skeletal muscle.

affected intestines are *taut*, then we must further conclude that the visceral afferents of the intestines are also connected with the motoneurons, whose axons innervate the abdominal muscles (*e* in Fig. 8-14), the *viscerosomatic* reflex. Warming of skin results in *inhibition of the intestinal motions* and thus reduces the pain. This effect is most certainly not direct but is transmitted as a nervous reflex. It is based on the segmental connection of the afferents of the thermoreceptors in the skin (*b* in Fig. 8-14) with the autonomic (sympathetic) efferents (*c* in Fig. 8-14) to the intestine (*cutaneovisceral* reflex).

These spinal autonomic reflexes occur particularly in patients whose spinal cord has been transected as a result of an accident (paraplegics). About two months after the accident, mechanical stimulation of the skin can provoke massive sweating and violent vascular reactions in the skin. The relay stations in the spinal cord that transmit these reactions are continuously inhibited in healthy persons by descending pathways.

Spinal micturition reflex. Some autonomic functions in the thoracic and the abdominal regions, such as the micturition mechanism, are controlled by spinal reflex centers that are relatively independent. The spinal nervous regulation of micturition will now be described as an example of these reflexes. This spinal regulation of the bladder exists in early infancy. When the CNS grows more mature as the person becomes older micturition is controlled by higher centers.

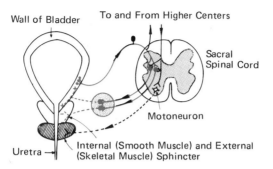

Wall of Bladder   To and From Higher Centers

Sacral
Spinal Cord

Motoneuron

Uretra   Internal (Smooth Muscle) and External
(Skeletal Muscle) Sphincter

Fig. 8-15. Nervous control of micturition. The parasympathetic spinal reflex arc is shown in red. For the sake of clarity, no interneurons are shown between afferent neuron and postganglionic neuron. The sympathetic innervation of the bladder muscles that originates in the first two lumbar segments has not been shown.

The wall of the bladder and its internal sphincter consist of smooth muscle. In addition, the bladder has a voluntarily controllable transverse-striated external sphincter muscle (see Fig. 8-15). In the denervated state the bladder empties itself once a certain degree of filling has been reached. The basic mechanism behind this autonomy of the micturition process, which takes place in the smooth muscles, was dealt with in Sec. 8.2 (see Fig. 8-6). Central nervous control of the bladder is superimposed on this autoregulation process. Nervous regulation is mediated by the parasympathetic system. The spinal reflex centers for this regulation are situated in the sacral cord (see Fig. 8-4).

The neurons involved in the autonomic nervous regulation of micturition are shown in red in Fig. 8-15. The bladder wall contains mechanoreceptors which measure the stretching of the wall. The afferents of these receptors are visceral. The excitation of the mechanoreceptors brought about by the filling of the bladder is transmitted by these visceral afferents to the sacral cord. In the sacral cord the activity of these afferents is transmitted to the preganglionic parasympathetic neurons (interneurons situated between preganglionic neurons and the mechanoafferents are not shown in Fig. 8-15). The activity is transmitted from the preganglionic neurons to the muscle of the bladder wall. This neuronal circuit is an *autonomic reflex arc*. As a result of the bladder filling, the smooth muscle of the bladder contracts in a reflex manner ("+" in Fig. 8-15), and the internal sphincter muscle around the urethra relaxes ("−" in Fig. 8-15), allowing the urine to be excreted.

In addition , the smooth muscles of the bladder are also innervated by sympathetic fibers that originate in the lumbar cord (not shown in

Fig. 8-15). These fibers have an effect on the smooth muscles of the bladder which is antagonistic to that of the parasympathetic system. It is a matter of dispute whether this innervation is of any great functional importance.

Micturition can also be controlled voluntarily. This is mediated by descending inhibitory and excitatory pathways that originate in higher centers in the brain stem and the cerebral cortex. As shown in Fig. 8-15, these pathways terminate on the preganglionic neurons and the motoneurons that innervate the striated external sphincter muscle of the bladder (Fig. 8-15).

Taken as a whole, the mechanism of micturition is *hierarchically* organized (organ level, spinal level, brain-stem level, cortical level). With each different level of control the emptying of the bladder can be adapted better to the needs of the organism. Regulation at the organ or the spinal level always brings about complete emptying when the bladder is full. Higher centers can intervene in this regulatory process and postpone micturition.

Preliminary remarks on the supraspinal control of circulation. The most important autonomic central nervous centers are situated in the *medulla oblongata*, which contains a large number of motor and sensory cranial nerve nuclei (for example, the vagal and the trigeminal nuclei). In addition, the medulla is traversed by many ascending and descending pathways (for example, the pyramidal pathway and the spinothalamic tract). The caudal part of the reticular formation is located in the spaces between the cranial nerve nuclei.

Respiration, circulation, and, to a great extent, the digestive process are regulated by the medulla. So far it has not been possible to pinpoint exactly where the autonomic centers are located in this mass of pathways, nuclei, and loose groups of neurons. The neurons that regulate circulation or respiration seem to be distributed over the entire medulla and embedded in the reticular formation. We can only say, for example, in which region of the medulla the neurons that promote circulation will most likely be found and in which region the inhibitory neurons will probably be located. Therefore, it only makes sense to talk of respiratory or cardiovascular *centers* in *functional* terms.

In the following, we will use the nervous regulation of the cardiovascular system as our example. This choice was made because more is known about the central nervous regulation of the cardiovascular system than about regulation of respiration and digestion. A further complicating factor in the case of respiration and digestion is that the somatic nervous system and hormonal factors also play an important role.

The circulatory system is the transportation system of the body. Oxygen and energy-rich substances are transported by the blood to the various organs (CNS, internal organs, muscles, and so on), and the waste products are removed. The cardiovascular system consists of the heart, the arteries, the veins, and the capillaries in the organs. With the exception of the capillaries, whose walls do not contain any smooth muscles, all parts of this system are autonomically innervated. In the arterial part of this system a mean blood pressure of about 100 mm Hg exists; this is about one-seventh of an atmosphere. The heart and the arterioles, in particular, play very important roles in maintaining this arterial blood pressure. The heart pumps the blood into the arterial system. The blood leaves the arterial system and enters the capillaries from the arterioles. The blood is transported back to the heart in the veins, where the pressure is about one-tenth of the arterial pressure. The walls of the veins are very soft and elastic, and the venous system contains about 80 percent of the total blood volume. The heart, the arterioles, and the veins are the most important autonomic effectors regulating circulation.

Inputs and outputs of the cardiovascular center. Figure 8-16 shows in diagrammatic form the most important components in the nervous control of circulation. The cardiovascular center is located in

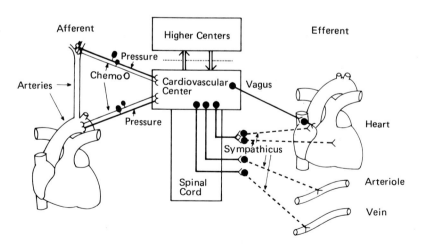

Fig. 8-16. Afferent and efferent neuronal connections of the cardiovascular center.

the medulla oblongata. This center functions even without the mod-
ifying influences of higher centers, for example, in the case of decerebrate animals. It receives information from the periphery through the
pressure receptors and the chemoreceptors in the aortic wall and in
the carotide bifurcation area (see Fig. 8-16, left). The *pressoreceptors*
measure the degree of stretching of the walls of the blood vessels
and consequently the mean and the pulsatile blood pressure. The
chemoreceptors measure the oxygen and the CO_2 tension in the arterial blood. The information from the pressoreceptors is normally
utilized more than that from the chemoreceptors for regulating the
circulation. The afferents of both receptors are visceral afferents.
When the arterial blood pressure is raised, the impulse frequency in
the afferents from the pressoreceptors increases; when the blood
pressure drops, the impulse frequency decreases.

The most important efferents of the cardiovascular center that
regulate circulation innervate the *heart*, the *arterioles*, and the *veins*
(Fig. 8-16, right). These efferents continuously transmit impulses to
their effectors and are *tonically* active. The heart beat and the contractile force of the heart are increased by the activity in the sympathetic
fibers. Parasympathetic fibers that run to the heart in the vagus nerve
(Fig. 8-4, 8-16) lower the heart rate. The arterioles and the veins are
innervated only by sympathetic fibers. As a result, the lumen of the
blood vessels is thus controlled solely by the magnitude of the activity
in these fibers. An increase in the sympathetic activity constricts the
blood vessels, and a decline dilates the vessels.

Regulation of blood pressure.   The cardiovascular center controls
the arterial blood pressure at a certain level in order to guarantee
adequate blood flow through the organs. The block diagram in Fig.
8-17 gives an overall view of the most important components of the
arterial blood pressure control system. The blood pressure is measured by the pressoreceptors in the aortic wall and carotid bifurcation
area and reported to the cardiovascular center via the afferents of the
receptors. If the blood pressure rises, the activity in the pressoreceptors increases; a drop in blood pressure is reported to the control
center by a decreased activity in the afferents from the pressure
receptors. The cardiovascular center adjusts an increased or decreased blood pressure to a normal level by varying the amount of
blood pumped by the heart in a certain period of time (*cardiac output*)
and the *diameter of the arterioles*. As mentioned in Sec. 8.3, the
cardiac output depends on the heart rate and the volume of blood
which the heart can pump out in a single contraction (stroke volume).
All three parameters—the diameter of the arterioles, the heart rate,

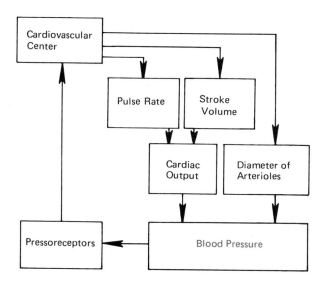

Fig. 8-17. Block diagram of the regulation circuit for controlling blood pressure. "Stroke volume" is the amount of blood pumped by the heart during one contraction. "Cardiac output" is the amount of blood pumped by the heart in a given amount of time (for example, 1 min).

and the stroke volume—are controlled by the sympathetic system, while the heart rate is controlled further by the parasympathetic system (see also Figs. 8-10 and 8-16).

If an animal's blood pressure is briefly increased by injecting sodium chloride solution into its arterial ciruclation, then in response the cardiac output is immediately reduced. This drop in the cardiac output is triggered centrally by a decrease in the activity of the sympathetic cardiac nerves and by an increase in the activity of the parasympathetic cardiac nerves. The arterioles in the organs are dilated by inhibition of the activity of the sympathetic fibers which innervate them. The effect of this is to boost the blood flow from the arterial system. As a result of these centrally triggered responses, the blood pressure immediately returns to normal.

Control of blood flow through the organs during muscular activity. The entire circulatory system is shown diagrammatically in Fig. 8-18A; on the right is the arterial system and on the left is the venous system; the left and the right ventricles of the heart are shown separately. In the center are shown the capillary regions of all the important organs (lungs, heart, brain, kidneys, intestines, skin, and skeletal muscles). The thickness of the arrows in the left and the right ventricles reflects the volume of blood pumped by the heart per unit

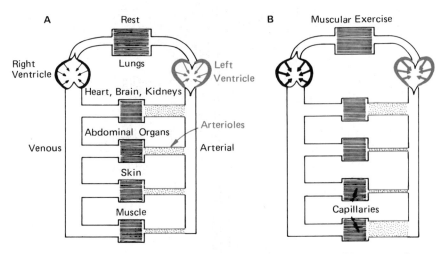

Fig. 8-18. Schematic view of the blood flow through the organs during resting conditions (A) and muscular exercise (B). The capillaries of the organs are shown in the center of the diagrams. The diameters of the arterioles (dotted red shading) indicate the amount of arterial blood flowing to the organs while at rest and during physical work.

time (cardiac output). The flow of blood through the organs is represented diagrammatically by the diameter of the arterioles (red).

Under *resting* conditions, about 45 percent of the cardiac output flows through the cardiac muscles, the brain, and the kidneys, 25 percent through the intestinal region, and 30 percent through the skin and the skeletal muscles. The magnitude of the various blood flows is indicated by the diameter of the arterioles in Fig. 8-18A (dotted red shading). When physical *work* is performed, the arterioles of the muscles performing the work are dilated by metabolic products which are generated in the muscle when energy-rich substances are broken down. As a result, more blood flows through the muscles; consequently more blood flows from the arterial system, and the blood pressure is lowered. This lowering of the blood pressure is reported to the cardiovascular center by the pressoreceptors (see Fig. 8-17).

Despite the increased flow through the muscle, the cardiovascular center maintains constant blood pressure by two mechanisms, as illustrated in diagrammatic form in Fig. 8-18B. First, the cardiac output (thick arrows in lumina of heart) increases, and more blood per unit time is pumped into the circulation. Second, the blood flow through the intestines and the skin is reduced by constriction of the arterioles (dotted red shading in Fig. 8-18B), while the blood flow through the vital organs—heart, brain, and kidneys—remains constant or increases slightly. As a result of these control measures—increase in cardiac output and reduction in blood flow through skin and intestines— considerably more blood flows through the muscles performing the work (see large diameter of arterioles in the muscles in Fig. 8-18B). During muscular exercise the sympathetic activity in the nerves leading to the heart and the blood vessels of the skin and the intestines is increased.

Q 8.12 Sketch the autonomic spinal reflex arc and indicate the afferent, the preganglionic, and the postganglionic neurons.

Q 8.13 "Stomach-ache" is usually caused by cramplike movements of the intestine. These pains can be eased by warming the skin of the abdomen (poultice). This effect is achieved because
  a. the intestine is directly warmed.
  b. the afferents of the thermoreceptors of the stimulated skin region are connected at the spinal level with sympathetic efferents that innervate the intestines.
  c. the parasympathetic centers in the medulla oblongata are stimulated in reflex fashion.
  d. the cutaneous blood vessels are dilated by the heat.
  e. a cutaneovisceral reflex arc exists at the segmental level.

Q 8.14 In response to a decrease in blood pressure the
  a. heart beat increases/decreases.
  b. diameter of the peripheral blood vessels increases/decreases.
  c. activity in the sympathetic cardiac nerves increases/decreases.
  d. activity in the pressoreceptors increases/decreases.

Q 8.15 The blood pressure of an animal is artificially lowered by letting it bleed. As a result the
  a. activity in the parasympathetic cardiac nerve is increased.
  b. activity in the afferents of the pressoreceptors is increased.
  c. arterioles are constricted.
  d. heart beat is lowered.
  e. activity in the sympathetic fibers that innervate the arterioles is increased.

8.5 The Hypothalamus. The Regulation of Body Temperature and Total Body Water

The previous section dealt with the simplest reflex centers at the spinal cord level and the medullary control of arterial blood pressure and blood flow through the organs. These autonomic reflex centers are subordinate to the hypothalamus, a phylogenetically old part of the

forebrain whose structure has remained relatively constant throughout the development of the vertebrates. In this respect the hypothalamus is quite different from other more recent parts of the forebrain,
such as the cerebral cortex and the cerebellum. Situated approximately in the "middle" of the brain, it assumes a central role as the
center that controls all the autonomic processes in the body. Therefore an animal without cerebrum is not particularly difficult to keep
alive, but an animal with no hypothalamus requires the utmost attention if it is not to die.

The various functions of the hypothalamus are dealt with in other
subject areas of physiology such as regulation of temperature and of
electrolyte balance, physiology of growth and maturation, and
physiology of the emotions. This diversity reflects the complexity of
the hypothalamic functions. However, all these functions have one
thing in common: they serve to keep the *internal conditions (milieu
interne)* of the body constant (*homeostasis*). In order to perform this
integrative function, the hypothalamus controls not only the
autonomic nervous system but also large parts of the *somatic* nervous
system and the *endocrine* system as well.

In the following, we will discuss the topographical position of the
hypothalamus and its most important afferent inputs and efferent
outputs. In order to make the regulatory character of its functions clear
we will use as examples the regulation of body temperature and the
total body water of the organism.

The topographical location of the hypothalamus. A medial view
of the brain in vertical cross section from front to rear is shown in Fig.
8-19A (from Fig. 7-10, p.207). (See small drawing alongside the anatomical sketch.) The region of the hypothalamus is marked in red. It is
located together with the thalamus *between* the cerebrum and the

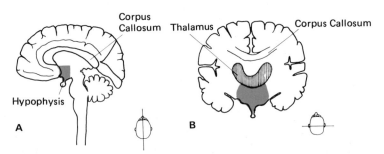

Fig. 8-19. Topographical location of the hypothalamus (red). The small
drawings at the bottom right in each case show the sections through the brain
in *A* and *B*.

mesencephalon. This region is therefore also called the *diencephalon*. For reasons of clarity the ventricles are not shown in this sketch. Figure 8-19*B* shows a cross section through the brain along a plane normal to that in Fig. 8-19*A*. The hypothalamus, marked red, is located below the thalamus as the word *hypo* implies.

The hypothalamus has a special relationship with the *hypophysis* (pituitary gland, Fig. 8-19*A, B)*. All the glands in the periphery of the body that produce hormones, for example, the thyroid and the sex glands are hormonally controlled by the hypophysis. The hypothalamus is functionally superior to the pituitary gland. It exerts nervous or hormonal control over the functions of the hypophysis; that is, it controls the amount of hypophysal hormones released.

The regulation of body temperature. Highly developed life is only possible if the internal conditions of the body, the *internal environment (milieu interne)* as they are collectively known, remain constant. These internal conditions include, for example, body temperature, blood-sugar concentration, and sodium-ion concentration in the blood. Maintenance of a constant internal environment is called *homeostasis*. Qualitatively one can make the following comparison. The body is permeated by the blood and the intercellular fluid which have a constant ion concentration, a constant carbon dioxide and oxygen tension, and so on. Thus, by analogy it may be said that the organism carries its environment with it much as an astronaut in his space suit or space capsule carries his life support system (oxygen, carbon dioxide, pressure, and so on) with him.

We will now describe the maintenance of a constant body temperature in detail to give an example of this higher level of hypothalamic control. In mammals it is essential for the functioning of the organism that body temperature be kept constant, since the rate of all chemical reactions in the body is temperature dependent, and the reactions occur optimally at 37 to 38 C.

When we consider the body temperature of warm-blooded animals, a distinction must be made between the temperature inside the body, for example, in the thorax or the brain *(core temperature)* and the temperature at the periphery of the body, for example, the limbs or the skin *(peripheral zone temperature)*. The peripheral zone temperature fluctuates considerably as a function of the ambient temperature (think of your cold fingers in winter), whereas the core temperature is held almost constant. The organism regulates its core temperature by two main mechanisms: the control of *heat production* and the control of *heat emission*. Heat is produced by the breakdown of energy-rich substances in the body (particularly fats and carbohydrates) and through muscular effort (muscular tremor). Increasing the metabolic activity thus results in *chemical* thermogenesis. Heat emission is regulated by control of the *cutaneous circulation.* The heat generated in the body is transported by the blood stream out to the skin and given off to the environment. The blood flow through the fingers, for example, can be varied by a factor of 1:600, and the amount of heat transported can be varied accordingly.

An important mechanism used for emitting heat, particularly in high ambient temperature conditions, is the *evaporation* of actively produced *sweat* at the surface of the body. Each liter of sweat that is completely evaporated removes a total heat energy of 580 kcal from the body, that is, approximately a quarter of the amount of energy that you take in each day with your food. In addition to these mechanisms, sensitivity to heat and cold elicits certain behavioral patterns, for example, the avoidance of extreme ambient temperatures, the choice of particular clothing, and so on, which can also be regarded in the broadest sense as control mechanisms for maintaining heat balance.

If the organism is to "know" when to remove heat and when to produce it, it must possess receptors (sensors) to measure the temperature. Sensors of this sort are located in the anterior portion of the hypothalamus and the skin of the organism. The sensors in the *anterior part of the hypothalamus* are specialized neurons (Fig. 8-20) which measure a rise in the core temperature *(heat receptors).* The sensors *in the skin* are *cold receptors* (Fig. 8-20) which record a lowering of the peripheral zone temperature. The latter temperature is reported to the center by these cold receptors before any drop in the core temperature can occur.

The posterior section of the hypothalamus controls, in particular, the production and the emission of heat (regulatory center in Fig. 8-20). On this center, information from the heat receptors in the

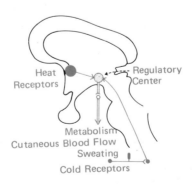

Fig. 8-20. Regulation of body temperature.

anterior part of the hypothalamus and from the cold receptors in the skin converges. If this part of the hypothalamus is destroyed, the organism may become poikilothermal. In other words, it can no longer keep its core temperature constant and independent of the ambient temperature.

Figure 8-21A shows a block diagram of the core temperature control system of the body. Figure 8-21B is a similar diagram of a modern thermostatically controlled central heating system. The body core temperature is maintained at 37 C, and the temperature in the room is held at 21 to 22 C. The inside thermometer in the house thus corresponds to the heat receptors in the hypothalamus. This inside thermometer measures the room temperature, and, similarly, the receptors in the anterior part of the hypothalamus measure the core temperature. The information from the heat receptors goes to another group of neurons in the posterior region of the hypothalamus (Fig. 8-20, regulatory center) that control the production and the emission of heat. In analogous fashion the information from the room thermometer is transmitted to the thermostat of the central heating system. If the room is too warm the heat output from the boiler is cut back. However, to lower the temperature in the room one can also open a window. In a very similar manner, when the core temperature is raised the metabolism is reduced, and the blood flow in the skin is increased. The greatest amount of heat can be removed from the body by sweating. There is no equivalent function in the control of room temperature. Both mechanisms of heat emmission—the increase in cutaneous blood flow and the secretion of sweat—are controlled by the sympathetic system. An increase in activity in the sweat gland fibers raises

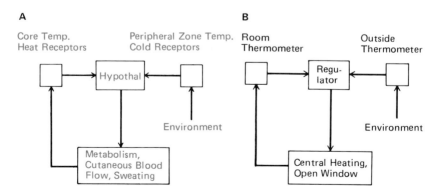

Fig. 8-21.   Block diagram of the regulation of body temperature (A) and room temperature (B). With the exception of "sweating," all the terms in or above the corresponding boxes in A and B are equivalent to each other.

the secretion of sweat. A decrease in the activity in the fibers that innervate the cutaneous blood vessels produces dilation of the vessels and increases the blood flow through the skin.

The control center in the posterior portion of the hypothalamus in addition receives information from the cold receptors in the skin. These receptors measure cooling of the skin; that is, they measure the peripheral zone temperature. The outside thermometer of a central heating system (Fig. 8-21B) operates in a fashion analogous to these cold receptors. The information from the outside thermometer is transmitted to the thermostat of the central heating system. If the ambient temperature drops, then the outside thermometer senses this, and the boiler heat output is set higher as a precaution because the heat losses in a room are greater when the ambient temperature is low. The information from the cold receptors is processed in analogous manner (Figs. 8-20 and 8-21A). If the ambient temperature drops, the metabolism of the organism is raised, and the cutaneous blood flow decreases. Adrenaline stimulates heat production by intervening directly in the chemical breakdown of fats and carbohydrates. This transmitter substance is released into the blood stream from the adrenal medulla.

Regulation of total body water. Like the body temperature, metabolism, water balance, and electrolyte balance are all controlled centrally by the hypothalamus. However in these cases, transmission from the regulatory center to the reacting organs is exclusively *hormonal*. The regulation of total body water will now be described using an example.

The ingestion of excessive amounts of liquid leads very rapidly to the production of urine. This rapid passing of the liquid demonstrates that the control system regulating the body water content is functioning successfully; this system protects the blood and the tissue fluids from becoming diluted. On the other hand, if nothing is drunk for a long time, urine production drops to a low level. The body tries to lose as little water as possible.

The way in which the total body water is regulated is illustrated in semidiagrammatic form in Fig. 8-22A. Sensors (receptors) which measure the degree of dilution of the blood are located in the anterior section of the hypothalamus. They are called *osmoreceptors*. These receptors are specialized neurons that react very sensitively to changes in the saline concentration of the surrounding tissue. The information from the osmoreceptors is transmitted to the hypophysis, which releases the hormone *vasopressin* into the blood. It is not known how many interneurons occur between the osmoreceptors and

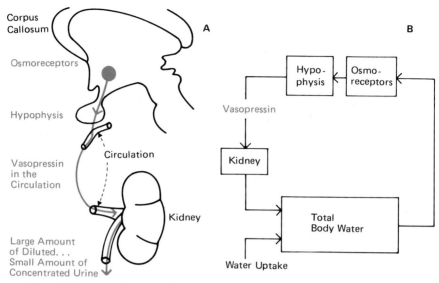

Fig. 8-22. Regulation of total body water. *A*: Semianatomical view. *B*: Block diagram representation.

the neurons that produce vasopressin. The *concentration* of vasopressin in the blood reports to the reacting organ, the kidney, how much water should be excreted. A high vasopressin concentration results in a small quantity of water being excreted; a low vasopressin concentration has the opposite effect; that is, a large quantity of water is excreted. Thus, if the total body water reaches a high level, only a small amount of vasopressin is released by the hypophysis, and a large amount of urine is excreted through the kidneys.

Figure 8-22*B* is a block diagram illustrating how the total body water is regulated and held constant when water is drunk. The ingestion of water results in a lowering of the saline concentration in the body. This drop is measured by the osmoreceptors and reported to the hypophysis. The hypophysis then reduces its release of vasopressin into the blood. The result is a reduction of the vasopressin concentration in the blood. The lower vasopressin concentration causes more water to be excreted by the kidneys. This in turn means that the total body water drops and returns to its old value. This hormonal control response takes place very rapidly and starts within 15 min. For a detailed description of the site of vasopressin production and of the parts of the kidney on which it acts, consult the relevant works published on hormone physiology and renal physiology.

Regulation of the endocrine glands (thyroid gland, suprarenal cortex, gonads, and so on), will not be discussed here in detail. The production of hormones by these glands is regulated by the hypothalamus by hormones from the hypophysis. In most cases even the connection between the hypothalamus and the hypophysis is hormonal (releasing factors). The feedback from the peripheral hormone glands to the hypothalamus takes place by measuring the concentration of the hormones of these glands in the blood.

The afferent and the efferent connections of the hypothalamus. The afferent (black arrows) and the efferent (red arrows) connections of the hypothalamus are shown in diagrammatic form in Fig. 8-23. These pathways stress the central functional position of the hypothalamus in the brain even more clearly than Fig. 8-19.

The hypothalamus is connected by efferent and afferent neuronal pathways with all higher and lower regions of the CNS. The two major higher regions are the limbic and the thalamocortical systems. The regions of the CNS below the hypothalamus are the brain stem and the spinal cord. The hypothalamus receives information from the environment through the five senses (hearing, smell, touch, sight, taste) and from the internal organs through the visceral afferents. To regulate total body water and body temperature, as mentioned above, the hypothalamus possesses specialized neurons that measure the salt concentration of the tissue and the temperature of the blood (core temperature). Also these parameters of the internal environment of

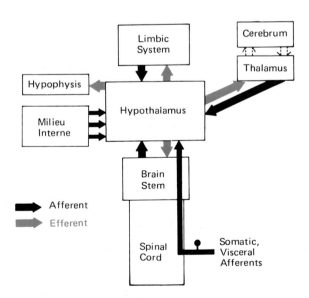

Fig. 8-23. Afferent and efferent connections of the hypothalamus. The afferent connections are shown in black, the efferent connections in red.

the organism are afferent inputs to the hypothalamus. The hypothalamus possesses special efferent outputs to the hypophysis. For the most part, these are *hormonal* in character. The release of hormones from the hypophysis is controlled by these connections. One of these hormones, namely, vasopressin, has been introduced in the description of total body water regulation.

Q 8.16 The hypothalamus is located
    a. beneath the thalamus.
    b. in the diencephalon.
    c. between the medulla oblongata and the cerebellum.
    d. in the cerebrum.
    e. between cerebrum and mesencephalon.

Q 8.17 During muscular exercise the body's heat production is raised. Which two ways are available to the body in order to keep its core temperature constant?
    a. Increase in sweat production.
    b. Reduction in cutaneous blood flow.
    c. Release of vasopressin into the blood stream.
    d. Increase in cutaneous blood flow.
    e. Release of adrenaline from the suprarenal cortex.

Q 8.18 When it is overheated, the body must give off heat to the environment. This emission of heat is controlled from the hypothalamus by
    a. neuronal mechanisms.
    b. hormonal mechanisms.
    c. neuronal and hormonal mechanisms.
    d. the sympathetic system.
    e. the parasympathetic system.

Q 8.19 Someone excretes 10 liters of urine per day and must therefore drink 10 liters of water per day. Where could the fault in the salt-water balance control system be located?
    a. The kidney can no longer excrete concentrated urine.
    b. The hypothalamus produces too much vasopressin.
    c. The water is being resorbed too quickly in the intestines.
    d. The vasopressin production is restricted as a result of a tumor in the hypothalamus.
    e. The sympathetic nervous system is overstimulated.

8.6 The Triggering and the Integration of Elementary Behavioral Patterns in the Hypothalamus

In the preceding section, the hypothalamus was shown to be the control center for many of the processes that take place in the organism. The internal conditions (internal environment) of the organism are held constant (homeostasis) by means of the hypothalamus. As a result, the organism is relatively independent of changes in the external environment. The hypothalamus is also the integrating center for elementary behavioral patterns: *defense behavior*, which comprises attack, self-defense, and flight (escape); *eating behavior*, which regulates food intake; and simple *reproductive (sexual) behavior*.

These aspects of behavior can be observed in an animal with an intact hypothalamus, but from which the entire cerebrum has been removed. Electrical stimulation of small, defined areas in the hypothalamus can also trigger such behavioral patterns. These attitudes may also be regarded as *homeostatic processes in a wider sense*, in that they enable the individual to exist in a hostile environment (defense behavior), guarantee intake of food (eating behavior), and serve to ensure propagation of the species (sexual behavior). In this section, we shall take the examples of eating and defense behavior to show that the elementary patterns consist of the coordination of individual somatic and autonomic reactions and that the hypothalamus integrates these reactions into a certain behavioral pattern.

Eating behavior.   The animal used in the following experiments is a conscious cat able to move around without restriction. Prior to the experiments a metal electrode was attached firmly to the head of the fully anesthetized cat. The tip of the electrode was positioned in the hypothalamus. If a certain group of cells in the lateral portion of the hypothalamus is stimulated through the electrode (100 stimuli per second for a duration of 10 sec), eating behavior is triggered. At the beginning of the experiment the animal is lying quietly, not paying attention to anything in particular. When the stimulus is applied the animal raises its head and looks alert. It stands up and starts to walk slowly around the room as if looking for something. It sniffs at the floor, goes to the food trough, and starts eating. This sequence of actions, from the first reaction to the final act of eating, is usually carried out within the 10-sec long series of stimuli. If the series of stimuli is interrupted, the cat stops eating. Repeating the stimulation produces the same behavioral pattern.

In order to check whether the eating behavior observed after electrical stimulation of the lateral hypothalamus also comprises autonomic reactions, the following were measured: blood pressure, intestinal movement, intestinal blood flow, and muscular blood flow (see Fig. 8-24, eating). Since it is difficult to measure the effect of hypothalamic stimulation on these parameters in the unrestricted animal, the cat was anesthetized. These four variables are continu-

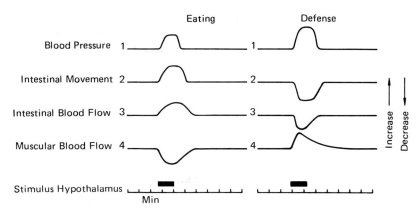

Fig. 8-24. Autonomic reactions during eating and defense behavior. Measurements 1 to 4 were obtained on an anesthetized cat. Small regions of the hypothalamus were stimulated with fine electrodes (black bar). (Modified from Folkow and Rubinstein: Acta physiol. Scand. **65,** 292, 1966.)

ously recorded in graph form in Fig. 8-24 (time axis at bottom of figure). The magnitude scales (ordinates) have been omitted for the sake of simplicity. Upward deviations indicate an increase in the measured values; downward deviations indicate a decline. Electrical stimulation of the region in the hypothalamus (heavy black line over time scale) from which eating behavior can be triggered causes the following changes in these variables: the blood pressure increases, the movements of the intestine increase, the blood flow through the intestine increases, and the blood flow through the skeletal muscles decreases. If the stimulation of the hypothalamus is terminated, the four variables return to their initial values. When the stimulation of the hypothalamus is repeated, the same autonomic changes are observed.

This redistribution of the blood flow through the organs in favor of the intestines is brought about by a lowering of the activity in the sympathetic fibers which innervate the intestinal blood vessels and an increase in the activity in the sympathetic fibers which constrict the blood vessels of the muscles (vasoconstrictors). The blood pressure increases as a result of an increase in the activity in the sympathetic cardiac nerves. The intestinal movements are induced by parasympathetic fibers which run in the vagus nerve. The eating behavior, which is observed after stimulation of the hypothalamus (standing up, walking around, bending down, chewing movements, and so on), is made up of the contractions of individual muscle groups; that is, it comprises motor reactions. The measurements in Fig. 8-24 (eating) show that during motor behavior, however, quite definite autonomic reactions also occur. The eating behavioral pattern thus includes both motor and autonomic reactions. Both reactions are coordinated in such a way that the organism is adjusted by the autonomic reactions to the process of *food intake*. The autonomic reactions that can be triggered by electrical stimulation of the hypothalamus are isolated fragments of the behavioral pattern that can be termed eating behavior. Some properties of this elementary behavior can also be observed in the decorticate animal whose limbic and thalamocortical systems have been removed. It can be said, therefore, that the hypothalamus is the *integration center* for this behavior.

Defense behavior. If the position of the tip of the electrode in the hypothalamus is varied by about 2 mm, then a completely different behavioral pattern can be triggered from this new area, namely, defense behavior. In purely descriptive terms this behavioral pattern consists of the elements of attack, self-defense, and flight (escape).

When the hypothalamus is stimulated, the animal, which was lying peacefully, suddenly becomes very alert. It gets up, arches its back, and starts to snarl, hiss, and paw. The digits of the paws are spread apart, and the claws are unsheathed. At the same time the animal's fur stands up, and the pupils open wide. All these reactions occur within a few seconds of hypothalamic electrical stimulation. These reactions can either terminate in a violent attack on the person conducting the experiment or the animal may try to run away. The behavior is accompanied by the secretion of saliva, urinating, and a tremendous increase in respiration. The behavior we have just described comprises some distinctly autonomic reactions which are triggered by an increase in activity in the sympathetic system (dilation of the pupils, fur standing up) or in the parasympathetic system (secretion of saliva, urinating). Behavioral attitudes with these autonomic characteristics are generally ascribed to the emotional expressions of *anger and fear* in man.

In order to measure the autonomic parameters shown in Fig. 8-24, the animal was again anesthetized. Figure 8-24 (defense) shows that the measurements change as follows during electrical stimulation (thick black line) of the region of the hypothalamus from which defense behavior can be triggered: the blood pressure increases, the movements of the intestine decrease, the blood flow through the intestines decreases, and the blood flow through the skeletal muscles increases. If we disregard the change in blood pressure, the measured autonomic reactions in the body change in opposite directions during the behavioral responses of "eating" and "defense." All the autonomic reactions during defense behavior can be explained by the increase in the activity in the sympathetic system. The intestinal movements and the blood flow through the wall of the intestine both decrease as a result of the increase in the sympathetic activity. The blood vessels of the skeletal muscles are said to be actively dilated by special sympathetic fibers whose transmitter substance to the smooth muscles of the blood vessels is said to be acetylcholine. As a result, the blood flow through the muscle increases. These changes in the autonomic parameters show that the reactive state of the organism during defense behavior is sympathetically based. This reactive state enables the organism to react in an optimum manner to threats from the environment. Defense behavior can be very easily triggered in the hypothalamic (decorticate) animal by painful and nonpainful stimulation of the skin. The hypothalamus is thus the *integration* center for the autonomic and the somatic reactions of elementary defense behavior.

It must be stressed here that such electrical stimulation of defined neuronal areas to trigger behavioral patterns is very nonspecific and crude in comparison with the precise coordination of autonomic and somatic reactions in a "natural" behavioral pattern. All the neurons in the area of the electrode tip are excited to an equal extent by the current, whereas when the behavioral response is "naturally" elicited the neurons are activated in specific patterns. In addition, one can object to the fact that these behavioral responses are triggered by stimulation of descending pathways; that is, that coordination actually takes place in higher centers. In fact, as already mentioned, to some extent these and other, particularly sexual, behavioral patterns can be triggered in decorticate animals with an intact brain stem by natural stimulation (for example, painful or nonpainful cutaneous stimuli). If the hypothalamus is separated from the brain stem in such animals, then it is no longer possible to generate these behavioral responses by either central electrical or natural stimulation.

The behavior patterns triggered in decorticate animals by natural stimulation follow a stereotyped course. When the stimulus is removed, they disappear immediately. The behavioral patterns can be triggered almost at will, as long as the decorticate animals stay alive. These patterns are not oriented to particular environmental situations, and it is highly unlikely that they correspond to particular emotional states or moods in the animal.

You have learned that the hypothalamus is subordinate to the *limbic system* (see Fig. 8-23). This system is phylogenetically the oldest part of the cerebrum and is completely covered by the newer parts of the cerebrum (frontal lobe, parietal lobe, temporal lobe, and so on). The limbic system probably generates the neurophysiological correlates of the emotions and regulates their relationships to certain environmental situations; that is, it is here that the schematic behavioral responses that are integrated and coordinated in the hypothalamus are triggered, differentiated, and adapted to the environmental situation. Thus, for example, an unusual but harmless stimulus (acoustic, visual, or tactile) at first triggers a reaction in the intact animal that is similar to the hypothalamic attack or flight response. If the stimulus, and the attack or the flight reaction does not materialize. On the other hand, a truly threatening situation is immediately recog- the stimulus, and the attack or flight reaction does not materialize. On the other hand, a truly threatening situation is immediately recognized when it occurs again—the animal remembers—and the corresponding defense response is triggered.

Q 8.20 During defense behavior (flight, attack)
    a. the cardiac output is increased.
    b. the digestion is promoted.
    c. the blood flow through the skeletal muscles is increased.
    d. the blood flow through the intestine is lowered.
    e. acetylcholine is released from the suprarenal cortex.

Q 8.21 A decorticate dog (cerebrum removed)
    a. can no longer maintain a constant body temperature.
    b. can remain alive if given the proper care.
    c. displays still some properties of feeding behavior.
    d. reacts defensively to strong cutaneous stimuli.
    e. dies because it can no longer regulate its circulation.

Q 8.22 Draw a diagram showing the changes, during eating behavior and defense behavior, in
    a. blood pressure.
    b. intestinal contractions.
    c. intestinal blood flow.
    d. muscle blood flow.

Answer Key

Chapter 1

Fig. 1-2: a, c, d = axon;
        b, f = dendrite;
        e, g = soma

Q 1.1:   b, c, e
Q 1.2:   c
Q 1.3:   See Fig. 1-1
Q 1.4:   See Fig. 1-4
Q 1.5:   b
Q 1.6:   a
Q 1.7:   a, b, c, e
Q 1.8:   c
Q 1.9:   b
Q 1.10: For nerve cells see
       Fig. 1-1.
       For connections
       between nerve cells
       see Fig. 1-4.
Q 1.11: Extracellular space,
       cerebrospinal fluid.
Q 1.12: Somatic afferents, motor
       efferents, autonomic
       efferents
Q 1.13: a, e
Q 1.14: a, b, d, e

Chapter 2

Q 2.1:   Fig. 2-5
Q 2.2: $K^+ = 20\text{-}100/1$
       $Na^+ = 1/5\text{-}15$
       $Cl^- = 1/20\text{-}100$
Q 2.3:   b, c reciprocal
Q 2.4:   a, c

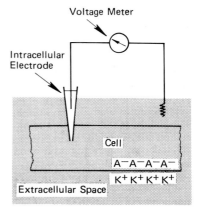

Fig. 2-5. Membrane charge and measurement of potential. Diagram to check answer to Q 2.1.

Q 2.5: $I_{Cl}/(E_{Cl}\text{-}E)$
Q 2.6: $E_{Na} = + 65mV$
Q 2.7:   b, c, d
Q 2.8:   b, c
Q 2.9:   a, d, e
Q 2.10: c
Q 2.11: Fig. 2-11
Q 2.12: b, c
Q 2.13: b
Q 2.14: b, d
Q 2.15: b
Q 2.16: Fig. 2-15
Q 2.17: a, c
Q 2.18: Fig. 2-18B
Q 2.19: b, c, d
Q 2.20: e
Q 2.21: d

Q 2.22: Fig. 2-21, bottom and
top curves
Q 2.23: c
Q 2.24: c, e
Q 2.25: a, b, c

Chapter 3

Q 3.1: a, b
Q 3.2: e
Q 3.3: c
Q 3.4: a, c
Q 3.5: c, d
Q 3.6: c, e
Q 3.7: d
Q 3.8: b
Q 3.9: c
Q 3.10: b
Q 3.11: a
Q 3.12: e
Q 3.13: b
Q 3.14: a, d
Q 3.15: b

Chapter 4

Q 4.1: b
Q 4.2: Neither. The two
excited populations
are summated.
Q 4.3: b, e
Q 4.4: c
Q 4.5: f
Q 4.6: b, c
Q 4.7: 12+15+3=30 msec
Q 4.8: a
Q 4.9: Nutritional reflexes: b,
d—Protective reflexes:
a, c, e, f
Q 4.10: c
Q 4.11: c
Q 4.12: b, e

Chapter 5

Q 5.1: Fig. 5-4
Q 5.2: b, d, f
Q 5.3: Fig. 5-2
Q 5.4: 1.) Myosin, 2.) Actin,
3.) Ca^{++}, 4.) <u>Adenosine
triphosphate</u> (Give in
any sequence)
Q 5.5: b, c
Q 5.6: c
Q 5.7: b, d
Q 5.8: c, d
Q 5.9: a,b,c
Q 5.10: b, c, d
Q 5.11: a, c
Q 5.12: b
Q 5.13: a, c
Q 5.14: d, e
Q 5.15: b, d

Chapter 6

Q 6.1: b
Q 6.2: a, d
Q 6.3: d
Q 6.4: d
Q 6.5: a) the muscle spindles
b) the tendon organs
Q 6.6: b, e, g
Q 6.7: b
Q 6.8: b, d, e
Q 6.9: c
Q 6.10: a
Q 6.11: d
Q 6.12: b, d, e
Q 6.13: d
Q 6.14: a, c
Q 6.15: a, d
Q 6.16: c
Q 6.17: e
Q 6.18: b, e
Q 6.19: b, e

Q 6.20: Neck afferents: a, b, c;
         Labyrinth: d
Q 6.21: a, d
Q 6.22: e
Q 6.23: b, d
Q 6.24: f
Q 6.25: f, there are no inhibitory
         synapses on the *den-*
         drites of the Purkinje
         cells
Q 6.26: b, d, e

Chapter 7

Q 7.1:   Mechano-, thermo-,
         chemo-, and
         photoreceptors
Q 7.2:   b, c
Q 7.3:   a, c, d
Q 7.4:   c
Q 7.5:   See Fig. 7-8
Q 7.6:   b, d
Q 7.7:   b, e
Q 7.8:   a, c, d, e
Q 7.9:   b, c
Q 7.10: d
Q 7.11: b, c
Q 7.12: b, c
Q 7.13: b, c
Q 7.14: a, b
Q 7.15: c

Q 7.16: a, c
Q 7.17: a, c

Chapter 8

Q 8.1:   a, c, d
Q 8.2:   b, c, d
Q 8.3:   c, e
Q 8.4:   b, c, d
Q 8.5:   a, d
Q 8.6:   a, d, e
Q 8.7:   b, c
Q 8.8:   a) seconds, b) 100,
         c) more slowly than
         d) later than
         e) the same
Q 8.9:   c, d
Q 8.10: a, d
Q 8.11: a, d
Q 8.12: see Fig. 8-13, left
Q 8.13: b, e
Q 8.14: a) increases,
         b) decreases,
         c) increases,
         d) decreases
Q 8.15: c, e
Q 8.16: a, b, e
Q 8.17: a, d
Q 8.18: a, d
Q 8.19: a, d
Q 8.20: a c, d
Q 8.21: b, c, d
Q 8.22: see Fig. 8-24

INDEX